CYTOKERATINS – TOOLS IN ONCOLOGY

Edited by **Gerhard Hamilton**

Cytokeratins – Tools in Oncology
Edited by Gerhard Hamilton

Published by InTech

Janeza Trdine 9, 51000 Rijeka, Croatia

Publishing Process Manager Martina Durovic

Technical Editor Teodora Smiljanic

Cover Designer InTech Design Team

Additional hard copies can be obtained from orders@intechopen.com

Cytokeratins – Tools in Oncology, Edited by Gerhard Hamilton
p. cm.
ISBN 978-953-51-0047-8

For EU product safety concerns:
IN TECH d.o.o., Prolaz Marije Krucifikse Kozulić 3, 51000 Rijeka, Croatia,
info@intechopen.com or visit our website at intechopen.com.

Meet the editor

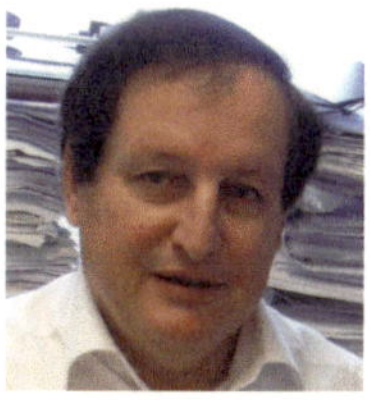

Dr. Gerhard Hamilton studied biochemistry at the University of Vienna, Austria. After finishing his doctoral thesis on Natural Killer cells he got a position in the research laboratories of the Department of Surgery at the University Medical School of Vienna and obtained the degree of associate professor in 1996. His scientific publications comprise the fields of organ transplantation, burn care, sepsis and oncology. Later on his research projects have focused on in vitro characterization of anticancer compounds such as novel platinum-based agents and titanocenes and respective mechanisms of drug resistance associated with cellular expression of relevant transporter proteins as well as changes in global gene expression. One special topic has been the investigation of diagnostic tests based on cytokeratin fragments in prostate and colorectal cancer patients revealing the applicability of the assays to prove residual tumor load. In addition, Dr. Hamilton has been the scientific coordinator of the "Ludwig Boltzmann Cluster of Translational Oncology" since 2006.

Contents

Preface

The present volume "Cytokeratins – Tools in Oncology" is a new addition to the Intech collection of books that aims at providing scientists and clinicians with a comprehensive overview of specific aspects of the latest research and current knowledge related to the application of cytokeratins in histology, cancer research and clinical diagnosis of tumors. For this purpose a series of research articles, clinical investigations and reviews that deal with the role of the most abundant cytokeratin types in normal and malignant tissues were included. This volume aptly adds to the other Intech titles in the field of oncology, particularly describing advances in cancer therapy, diagnosis and treatment of individual tumor entities as well as the important topic of cancer stem cells.

The participating authors shared their expertise about the multiple functions of cytokeratins in organization of the intermediary filaments in normal intestine and liver as well as microfold L cells and, furthermore, the usability of cytokeratins 7, 8, and 20 in tumor diagnosis. Epithelial to mesenchymal transition as a mechanism important in pathogenesis is touched in another chapter, followed by several articles discussing the assessment of cytokeratins in disseminated tumor cells and as response markers during chemotherapy. Our group published reports on the use of cytokeratin fragments in prostate cancer patients undergoing intermittent androgen suppression in the late nineties and it was fascinating to observe the continuative development of anti-cytokeratin reagents as diagnostic and possible predictive tools available in the form of refined assays providing highly valuable means to detect the presence of disseminated tumor cells and minimal residual disease in cancer patients. This book is therefore destined to all cancer researchers and therapists who want to understand the diagnostic use of cytokeratins in histology and especially to tackle the challenge of finding residual tumor cells in patients, either circulating in the blood or residing hidden in niches, that may lead to tumor recurrence and qualify patients for a more aggressive anticancer therapy.

As editor of this book, I would like to acknowledge the significant efforts made by all of the contributing authors and the entire editorial team in publishing of this work. I would like to dedicate this book to the "Ludwig Boltzmann Society" and, in particular, to Prof. Dr. Gerhard Baumgartner whose long-standing support has allowed for the successful realization of many scientific projects. Last but not least, I would like to thank my wife for her personal support and great patience at all times.

Gerhard Hamilton, PhD
Ludwig Boltzmann Cluster of Translational Oncology, Vienna, Austria

Part 1

Expression of Cytokeratins in Nonmalignant Tissue

1

The Expression of Cytokeratins in Bovine Intestinal Microfold (M) Cells

Takashi Kanaya[1], Tetsuya Hondo[1], Kohtaro Miyazawa[1], Michael T. Rose[2] and Hisashi Aso[1]
[1]*Tohoku University*
[2]*Aberystwyth University,*
[1]*Japan*
[2]*UK*

1. Introduction

The mucosal surface of the gut is exposed to a variety of foreign antigens and microorganisms, some of which are potentially harmful for the host. To protect against the risk of infection, the intestinal mucosa has developed specialized organized lymphoid tissues and epithelial cells. The gut-associated lymphoid tissues (GALT) including Peyer's patches (PPs) are major inductive sites for intestinal immunity. Different from other peripheral lymphoid tissues, GALT lacks afferent lymphatics, and directly samples mucosal antigens across the epithelial barrier to initiate antigen-specific immune responses. This task is accomplished by specialized epithelial cells within the follicle-associated epithelium (FAE) covering the lymphoid follicles of GALT known as microfold (M) cells.

M cells possess a high capacity for phagocytosis and transcytosis, and these functions allow the rapid transport of antigens into the underlying lymphoid tissues, especially antigen-presenting cells. Antigens are then presented to T cells that support B-cell activation, resulting ultimately in the generation of IgA-producing plasma cells. Thus, M-cell-mediated antigen transport is important for the initiation of mucosal immune responses (Kraehenbuhl and Neutra, 2000; Neutra et al., 1996; Neutra et al., 2001). In order to express their specialized functions including phagocytosis and transcytosis, M cells exhibit unique morphologies that differ from the surrounding absorptive enterocytes. M cells lack a dense microvilli brush border structure, though they do possess shorter and irregular microvilli on their apical surface. On the basolateral side, a pocket-like invagination of the plasma membrane is formed to house lymphocytes and antigen-presenting cells (Neutra et al., 1996).

These morphological features of M cells have an effect on the composition of the cytoskeletal proteins within the cell, such as actin-containing microfilaments, intermediate filaments and their associated proteins. For example, the lack of a brush border in M cells is reflected in the cellular localization of the actin and villin, resulting in unusual staining patterns of these proteins in M cells of mice and calves, as actin and villin are essential proteins for microvilli formation (Kanaya et al., 2007; Kerneis et al., 1996). In addition to the abnormal cellular localization of actin and actin-related proteins, some investigators have demonstrated that intermediate filament proteins such as vimentin and cytokeratins can be used as immunohistochemical markers for M cells. Gebert *et al.* have shown that CK18 is a sensitive marker for porcine M cells (Gebert et al., 1994) while vimentin is selectively expressed in rabbit M cells (Jepson et al., 1992). M cells in rats are detected by monoclonal antibodies raised against CK8 (Rautenberg et al., 1996). These preferential expressions of intermediate filaments in M cells indicate the substantial roles of CKs and vimentin in M cell morphology and function.

In this chapter, we introduce a number of experiments that we have done with respect to the expression of CK18 in bovine M cells. And we further discuss the relationship between the expressions of CKs and the development and apoptosis of bovine intestinal M cells.

2. Material and methods

In this study, we performed several histological and electron microscopical analyses. The monoclonal antibodies for immunohistochemistry are summarized in Table 1. The detailed procedures have been described in our previous reports (Hondo et al., 2011; Miyazawa et al., 2006).

3. Results

3.1 Localization of M cells in FAE of jejunum and ileum PPs

The distribution and size of PPs in ruminants, including cattle, have several unusual features. PPs in the jejunum resemble those of other mammalian species. In addition to these jejunal PPs, however, ruminants possess another type of PPs in the ileum. These ileal PPs make up about 15% of the length of the small intestine, and are thought to be mature before birth and involute at a young age, in a similar way to the thymus gland (Beyaz and Asti, 2004; Landsverk, 1979, 1984; Reynolds and Morris, 1983). In order to observe the localization of bovine M cells in both jejunal and ileal PPs, we examined the ultrastructure of the FAE by scanning electron microscopy (SEM) in 13 weeks old calves. In jejunal PPs, M cells were randomly distributed in the FAE as for other species (Figure 1). On the other hand, the FAE of ileal PPs were almost filled with M cells having irregular microvilli (Figure 1). These observations are consistent with previous reports (Kanaya et al., 2007; Landsverk, 1984).

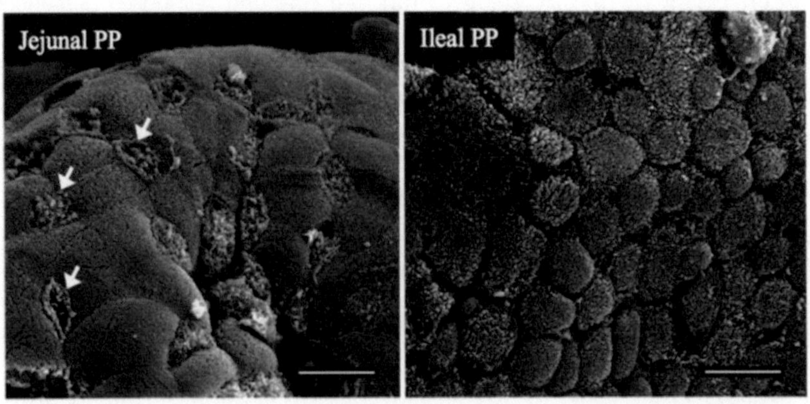

Fig. 1. Scanning electron microscopy (SEM) of follicle-associated epithelium (FAE) in bovine Peyer's patches (PPs).

The specimens of PPs were fixed with 2.5% glutaraldehyde and coated with platinum-palladium for SEM analysis. SEM shows the distribution of M cells in the FAE of jejunal PPs and ileal PPs. Arrows show M cells possessing irregular and sparse microvilli in jejunal PPs. The FAE of ileal PPs is filled with M cells. Bars = 10 μm.

3.2 Expression of CK18 in bovine M cells

As described above, some intermediate filament proteins, such as CK8, CK18, and vimentin, are known to be marker for M cells in the intestine. Therefore, we investigated the expressions of these proteins in bovine PPs (see table 1). As a result of this, we identified that several monoclonal antibody clones for CK18 were preferentially stained in the FAE and crypts of both jejunal and ileal PPs (Figure 2, 3A and B). CK20 was detected strongly in both the villous epithelium and FAE, but not in the crypts. In contrast, CK7, CK8 and CK19 could not be detected in the whole of the small intestinal epithelium, and vimentin was only detected in the stromal cells of subepithelial tissues (Figure 2 and Table 1). The positive CK18 signal in the FAE of jejunal and ileal PPs was similar to the distribution of M cells recognized by SEM. In order to confirm the expression of CK18 in bovine M cells, we investigated the ultrastructure of CK18-positive cells in the FAE. In jejunal FAE, CK18-positive cells had irregular and sparse microvilli and pocket-like structures containing lymphocytes (Figure 3C and E). In the sections of ileal FAE, we clearly observed that CK18-positive cells had broader microfolds on their apical surface, and CK18-negative cells had dense microvilli (Figure 3D and F). In addition to the preferential expression of CK18 in M cells, CK18 was also detected in the crypts (Figure 2). Therefore, we investigated the proliferative activity of CK18-positive cells in the crypt using the mirror section technique. A couple of mirror sections revealed that all Ki-67 positive proliferative cells in the crypt were positive for CK18 (Figure 4). These results suggest that CK18 is a marker for M cells in the both jejunal and ileal FAE, and proliferative cells in the crypts of the bovine small intestine.

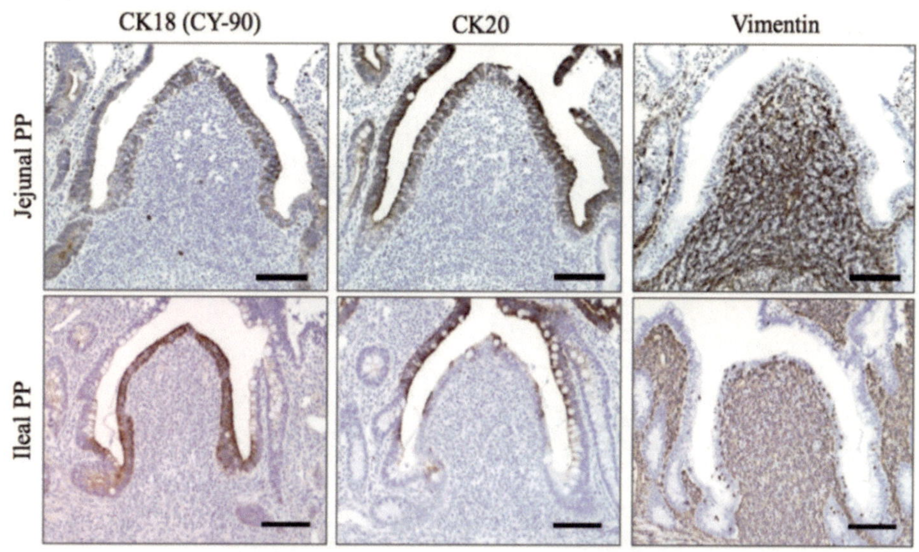

Fig. 2. Expression of cytokeratins and vimentin in bovine PPs.

The sections were immunostained with anti-cytokeratin (CK) 18 (CY-90), anti-CK20 and anti-vimentin monoclonal antibodies. Bars = 100 μm.

Specificity	Isotype	clone#	Dilution	Staining patterns
Pan-CK	Mouse IgG_1	C-11	1: 2000	M cells, crypt
CK7	Mouse IgG_1	RCK105	1: 1000	N. D.
CK8	Mouse IgM	35βH11	Ready to use	N. D.
CK18	Mouse IgG_1	CY-90	1: 1000	M cells, crypt
CK18	Mouse IgG_1	Ks-B17.2	1: 1000	M cells, crypt
CK18	Mouse IgG_1	CK5	1: 500	M cells, crypt
CK19	Mouse IgG_{2a}	A53-B/A2	1: 100	N. D.
CK20	Mouse IgG_{2a}	Ks20.8	1: 2	Villus epithelium, FAE enterocytes
Vimentin	Mouse IgG_{2a}	VIM 3B4	Ready to use	Sub epithelium
Ki67	Mouse IgG_1	MIB-1	1: 100	Proliferative cells

Table 1. The list of monoclonal antibodies against intermediate filaments proteins.

The specificity, isotypes, clone numbers, dilution for immunostaining and staining patterns in bovine PPs of antibodies against intermediate filament proteins are summarized. N. D. means "Not detectable".

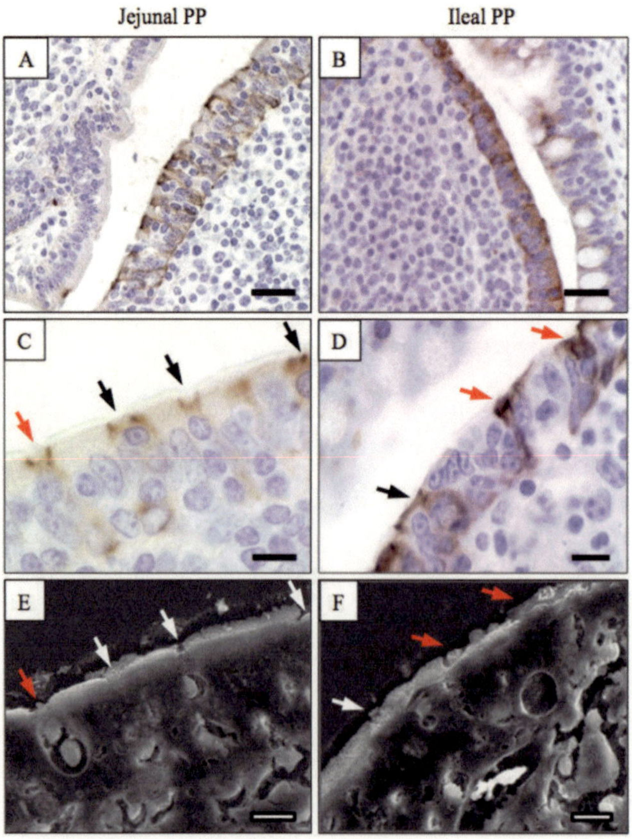

Fig. 3. Ultrastructure of CK18-positive cells in bovine PPs.

CK18-positive cells showed M-cell like distribution in the FAE of jejunal and ileal PPs (A and B). A couple of mirror sections were used for the identification of CK18-positve cells. One section was stained with anti-CK18 (CY-90) monoclonal antibody (C and D). The other was fixed with glutaraldehyde, treated with tannic acid, and coated with platinum-palladium for SEM analysis (E and F), respectively. Arrows show identical cell types. Bars = 30 µm (A and B) and 10 µm (C-F).

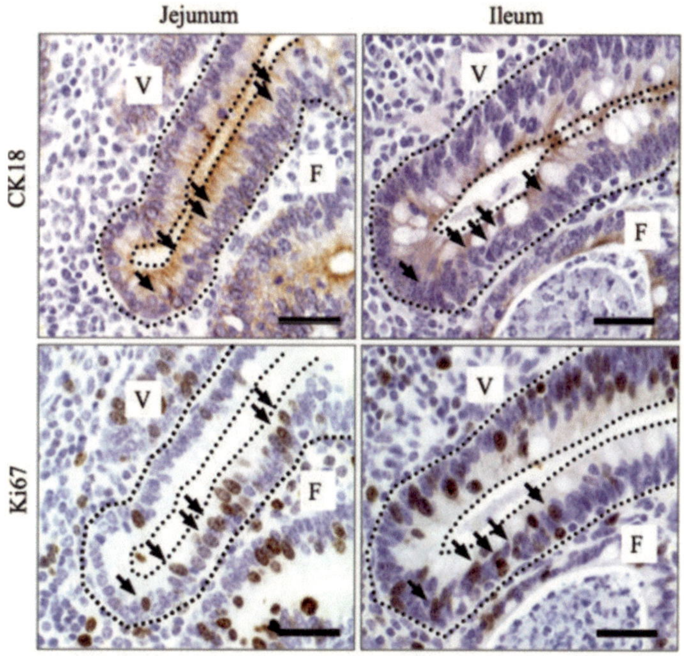

Fig. 4. Localization of CK18-positive cells in the crypts

For the identification of CK18-positive cells in the crypts, we prepared a couple of mirror sections of crypts containing villous epithelium (V) and FAE (F), which were immunostained with anti-CK18 monoclonal antibody or anti-Ki67 monoclonal antibody, a marker of proliferation. Arrows show Ki67-positive cells. Dotted lines show the epithelial cells of the crypts. Bars = 30 µm.

3.3 The relationship of CK18 and CK20 in the bovine FAE

CK20 was observed not only throughout the epithelial cells lining villous epithelium, but also in the partial cells of the FAE (Figure 2). These results demonstrate that both CK18 and CK20 are co-expressed in the FAE-crypt axis. Therefore, we investigated the expression of these CKs in the FAE-crypt axis by dual staining of CK18 and CK20. As described above, the preferential expression of CK18 was observed in the M cells of the FAE and proliferative cells in the crypts. On the other hand, CK20 positive signals were exclusively observed in the CK18-negative cells including the partial of the FAE cells and the whole of villous epithelial cells (Figure 5A-D). These results indicate that proliferative cells in the crypts exchange CK18 for CK20 once above the mouths of crypts when they have moved to the villi, whereas M cells continue expressing CK18 during their movement from the crypt to the FAE.

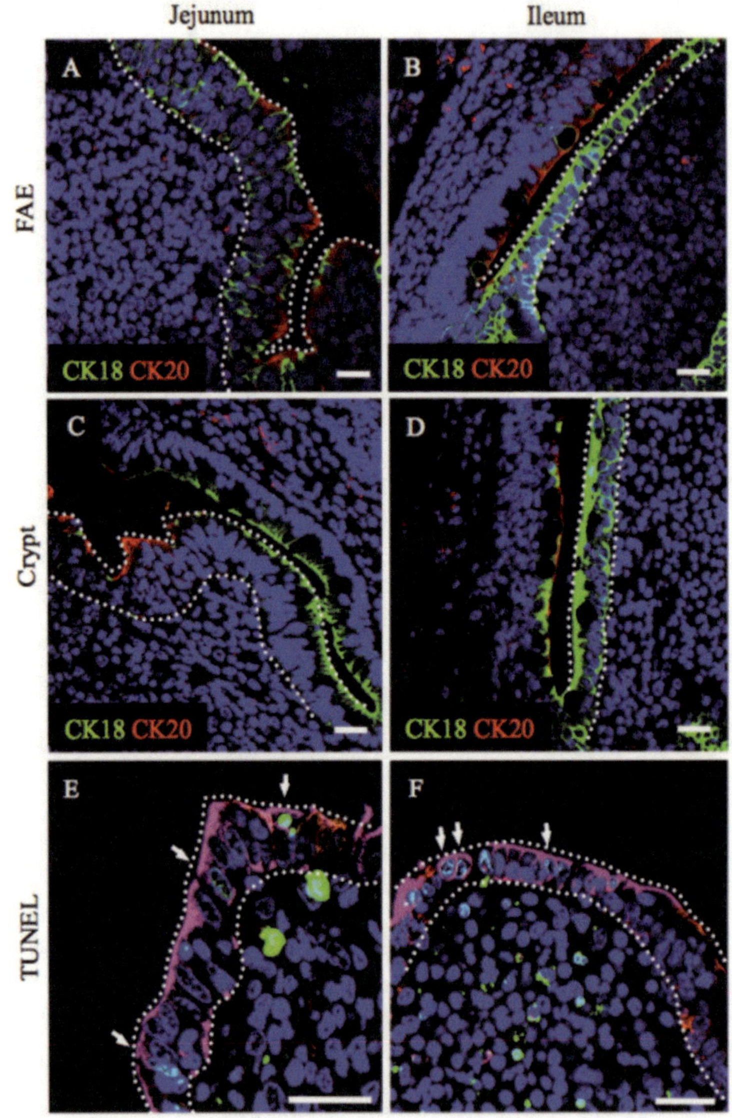

Fig. 5. Localization of CK18-, CK20-, and TUNEL-positive cells in the jejunum and ileum.

Jejunum and ileum sections were dual immunostained with anti-CK18 (IgG_1) and CK20 (IgG_{2a}) monoclonal antibodies. CK18 and CK20 were visualized by goat Alexa 488 anti-mouse IgG_1 (green) and by goat Alexa 594 anti-mouse IgG_{2a} (red) antibodies (A-D). Apoptotic cells were detected with the Dead End Fluorometric terminal deoxynucleotidyl-transferase-mediated deoxyuridine-triphosphate-biotin nick-end labeling (TUNEL) system. The sections of jejunal and ileal FAE were stained using the TUNEL method and immunostained with anti-CK18 (IgG_1) and CK20 (IgG_{2a}) monoclonal antibodies. CK18 and CK20 were visualized by goat Alexa 546 anti-mouse IgG_1 (orange) and by goat Alexa 647 anti-mouse IgG_{2a} (magenta) antibodies (E and F). Arrows show TUNEL-positive cells. Dotted lines show FAE. Bars = 10 µm.

3.4 Apoptosis of bovine M cells

It has been reported that M cells possibly transdifferentiate into enterocytes before exclusion from the FAE apex in the porcine small intestine (Miyazawa et al., 2006). To investigate these events for bovine intestinal M cells, we performed a triplicate CK18 and CK20, and TUNEL staining. The TUNEL-positive apoptotic cells were observed at the apical region of villi in both the jejunum and ileum (data not shown, see Hondo et al., 2011). We could also see TUNEL-positive signals in the apex of both jejunal and ileal FAE; however, TUNEL-positive apoptotic cells were only observed in CK20-positive cells (Figure 5E and F), indicating that only enterocytes could undergo apoptosis. Moreover, we quantified the cells that were positive for CK18, CK20 and apoptosis in the crypt-villus axis to evaluate the possibility that M cells transdifferentiate into enterocytes. The sections containing TUNEL-positive cells were selected, and the distance from the mouth of the crypt to the apex of half of the FAE was divided into thirds: lower, peripheral and apical regions. The proportions of CK18-positive cells in the lower region were 45 and 96% in the jejunal and ileal FAE, respectively, and these rates decreased to 21 and 57% at the apical regions of the FAE. On the other hand, the number of CK20-positive cells gradually increased from the lower region to the apex (Table 2). These data suggest that bovine M cells, positive for CK18, may transdifferentiate into CK-20 positive enterocytes before they undergo apoptosis at the apex of the FAE.

Regions	Marker	Cell No.	TUNEL+ Cell	CK18 (%)/CK20 (%)
Jejunum (n = 13)				
Total cell no./half FAE		91.5 ± 11.9		
Lower	CK18	13.9 ± 2.3	0	45.2 ± 54.8
	CK20	16.8 ± 2.4	0	
Peripheral	CK18	12.1 ± 3.0	0	39.2 ± 60.8
	CK20	18.4 ± 2.2	0	
Apical	CK18	6.5 ± 2.3	0	21.3 ± 78.7
	CK20	23.8 ± 3.1	1.9 ± 0.8	
Ileum (n = 10)				
Total cell no./half FAE		58.7 ± 6.2		
Lower	CK18	19.1 ± 1.8	0	96.1 ± 3.9
	CK20	0.8 ± 1.0	0	
Peripheral	CK18	18.3 ± 1.8	0	93.8 ± 6.2
	CK20	1.3 ± 1.7	0	
Apical	CK18	11.0 ± 2.6	0	57.2 ± 42.8
	CK20	8.2 ± 2.5	3.1 ± 0.7	

Table 2. Configurational comparison of CK18 and CK20-positive cells in jejunal and ileal FAE.

Results for cell no. and terminal deoxynucleotidyl-transferase-mediated deoxyuridine-triphosphate-biotin nick-end labeling (TUNEL)-positive cells are expressed as means ± SD; n, no. of cells. Results for cytokeratin (CK) 18/CK20 are expressed as the ratio of the proportion of CK18-positive cells to that of CK20-positive cells in each region of the FAE. The sections from jejunal and ileal follicle-associated epithelium (FAE) were stained with anti-CK18 and anti-CK20 monoclonal antibodies and TUNEL. The sections containing TUNEL-positive cells were selected. One-half of the FAE was divided into thirds (lower region, from the mouth of crypt to the peripheral region; peripheral region, middle third of the FAE; and apical region, upper third of the FAE).

3.5 The expression of CK18 and CK20 in duodenum and colon

We investigated the expression patterns of CK18 and CK 20 in the duodenum and colon. In the duodenum, CK18 was also detected in the crypt. These CK18-positive cells moved to the villi and gradually changed CK18 for CK20 at the mouth of the crypts as observed in the crypt-villus axis of the jejunum and ileum (Figure 6). Besides this, prominent expression was also observed in Brunner glands of the duodenum (Figure 6A and B). In the colon, CK18-positive cells were observed in almost all crypt cells, and this was changed for the expression of CK20 at the mouth of the crypt (Figure 6C and D). This observation is similar to that for the mouse, indicating that CK18 and CK20 expression patterns are conserved across these species, except for the expression of CK18 in bovine M cells.

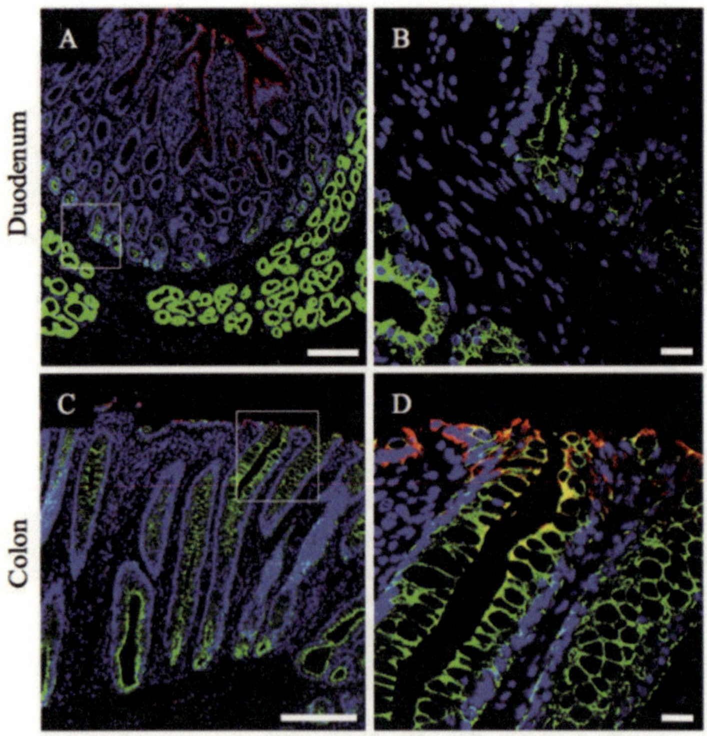

Fig. 6. CK18 and CK20 expression in the duodenum and colon.

Sections of duodenum (A and B) and colon (C and D) were dual immunostained with anti-CK18 (IgG_1) and anti-CK20 (IgG_{2a}) monoclonal antibodies. CK18 and CK20 were visualized by Alexa 488 goat anti-mouse IgG_1 (green) and Alexa 594 goat anti-mouse IgG_{2a} (red) antibodies, respectively. B and D are higher magnification of the boxes in A and C, respectively. Bars = 200 µm (A and C) and 10 µm (B and D).

4. Conclusions

We have demonstrated that CK18 is expressed in bovine M cells, providing a useful tool for the detection of bovine intestinal M cells. Unlike some other mammals, ruminants develop two types of PPs in the jejunum and ileum, respectively, and both PP types possess different phenotypes for FAE and M cells. On the basis of this, we carefully observed the expression of CK18 in these M cells, and identified that both jejunal and ileal M cells were clearly detectable by immunohistochemistry of CK18. This method enabled us to detect an entire set of bovine M cells, and this will contribute to ongoing investigations of bovine M-cell differentiation and function.

Intestinal epithelial cells are well known to derive from stem cells located at the bottom of crypts (Barker and Clevers, 2010). Although M cells are an intestinal epithelial cell type, their origin has not been clarified; M cells directly differentiate from intestinal stem cells, or mature enterocytes, and convert into M cells under the influence of lymphocytes or microorganisms (Kerneis et al., 1997; Savidge et al., 1991). Recent analyses seem to support that M cells directly differentiate from stem cells, for example, Clevers *et al.* have shown that M cells derive from Lgr5-positive stem cells at the bottom of the crypt in the Lgr5-reporter mouse (Barker and Clevers, 2010). In the bovine intestine, proliferative cells, including the stem cell compartment and M cells, express CK18, indicating that CK18 expressed in immature cells continues into the M-cell lineage. Although these unique expression patterns are bovine specific, this aspect may help with clarifying the biological function of CK18 in intestinal epithelial cells. Our studies also confirm the possibility that M cells may transdifferentiate into enterocytes before apoptosis by examining the expression patterns of CK18 and CK20 in the crypt-FAE axis. Similar phenomena have been observed in murine and porcine M cells (Miyazawa et al., 2006; Sierro et al., 2000), indicating that this transdifferentiation of M cells into enterocytes is conserved for the M-cells of some species.

M cells are thought to be involved in the infections of various pathogens, such as pathogenic bacteria, viruses or prions (Brayden et al., 2005; Clark et al., 1998; Heppner et al., 2001; Takakura et al., 2011). In addition, we have recently demonstrated that bovine M cells possess a higher capacity for transporting the transmissible spongiform encephalopathies (TSE) agent than enterocytes *in vitro* (Miyazawa et al., 2010), suggesting a risk of bovine M cells as the entry site for some pathogens. The detection of bovine M cells by CK18 will contribute to the *in vivo* examination of the infectious mechanisms of various pathogens in the bovine intestine.

It is well known that different types of cells and tissues are characterized by the specific composition of their intermediate filaments. In the small intestine, CK7, CK8, CK18, CK19 and CK20 are expressed in epithelial cells (Flint et al., 1994; Kucharzik et al., 1998; Zhou et al., 2003). The subgroup of cytokeratins might serve as potent differentiation markers, because the diverse expression patterns of cytokeratins are correlated with epithelial differentiation (Moll et al., 1982). In the murine intestine, several CKs exhibit distinct expression patterns: CK7 and CK18 are strongly expressed in the crypt region, whereas

CK20 is expressed in differentiated epithelial cells lining the villi (Zhou et al., 2003). In this study, we have investigated the expression of various CKs in the bovine intestine, and demonstrated that CK18 and CK20 are expressed in the bovine intestinal tract. The expression of CK18 in the crypts and that of CK20 in villi were very similar to the expression patterns of mice. These conserved expression patterns of CK18 and CK20 indicate that these CKs are fundamental cytoskeletal proteins in intestinal epithelial cells. In addition, it has been reported that CK20 is important for keratin filament organization, and that both CK18 and CK20 have functional redundancy (Zhou et al., 2003). We observed that CK18 and CK20 did not co-localize throughout the FAE- or villus-crypt axis, implying important functional roles for CK18 and CK20 in the keratin filament formation in each compartment.

5. Acknowledgment

This study was supported by a Grant-in-Aid for Scientific Research (21380170) from the Ministry of Education, Culture, Sports, Science and Technology, and BSE Control Project from the Ministry of Agriculture, Forestry and Fisheries.

6. References

Barker, N., and Clevers, H. (2010). Leucine-rich repeat-containing G-protein-coupled receptors as markers of adult stem cells. Gastroenterology *138*, 1681-1696.

Beyaz, F., and Asti, R.N. (2004). Development of ileal Peyer's patches and follicle associated epithelium in bovine foetuses. Anat Histol Embryol *33*, 172-179.

Brayden, D.J., Jepson, M.A., and Baird, A.W. (2005). Keynote review: intestinal Peyer's patch M cells and oral vaccine targeting. Drug Discov Today *10*, 1145-1157.

Clark, M.A., Hirst, B.H., and Jepson, M.A. (1998). M-cell surface beta1 integrin expression and invasin-mediated targeting of Yersinia pseudotuberculosis to mouse Peyer's patch M cells. Infect Immun *66*, 1237-1243.

Flint, N., Pemberton, P.W., Lobley, R.W., and Evans, G.S. (1994). Cytokeratin expression in epithelial cells isolated from the crypt and villus regions of the rodent small intestine. Epithelial Cell Biol *3*, 16-23.

Gebert, A., Rothkotter, H.J., and Pabst, R. (1994). Cytokeratin 18 is an M-cell marker in porcine Peyer's patches. Cell Tissue Res *276*, 213-221.

Heppner, F.L., Christ, A.D., Klein, M.A., Prinz, M., Fried, M., Kraehenbuhl, J.P., and Aguzzi, A. (2001). Transepithelial prion transport by M cells. Nat Med *7*, 976-977.

Hondo, T., Kanaya, T., Takakura, I., Watanabe, H., Takahashi, Y., Nagasawa, Y., Terada, S., Ohwada, S., Watanabe, K., Kitazawa, H., *et al.* (2011). Cytokeratin 18 is a specific marker of bovine intestinal M cell. Am J Physiol Gastrointest Liver Physiol *300*, G442-453.

Jepson, M.A., Mason, C.M., Bennett, M.K., Simmons, N.L., and Hirst, B.H. (1992). Co-expression of vimentin and cytokeratins in M cells of rabbit intestinal lymphoid follicle-associated epithelium. Histochem J *24*, 33-39.

Kanaya, T., Aso, H., Miyazawa, K., Kido, T., Minashima, T., Watanabe, K., Ohwada, S., Kitazawa, H., Rose, M.T., and Yamaguchi, T. (2007). Staining patterns for actin and villin distinguish M cells in bovine follicle-associated epithelium. Res Vet Sci *82*, 141-149.

Kerneis, S., Bogdanova, A., Colucci-Guyon, E., Kraehenbuhl, J.P., and Pringault, E. (1996). Cytosolic distribution of villin in M cells from mouse Peyer's patches correlates with the absence of a brush border. Gastroenterology *110*, 515-521.

Kerneis, S., Bogdanova, A., Kraehenbuhl, J.P., and Pringault, E. (1997). Conversion by Peyer's patch lymphocytes of human enterocytes into M cells that transport bacteria. Science *277*, 949-952.

Kraehenbuhl, J.P., and Neutra, M.R. (2000). Epithelial M cells: differentiation and function. Annu Rev Cell Dev Biol *16*, 301-332.

Kucharzik, T., Lugering, N., Schmid, K.W., Schmidt, M.A., Stoll, R., and Domschke, W. (1998). Human intestinal M cells exhibit enterocyte-like intermediate filaments. Gut *42*, 54-62.

Landsverk, T. (1979). The gastrointestinal mucosa in young milk-fed calves. A scanning electron and light microscopic investigation. Acta Vet Scand *20*, 572-582.

Landsverk, T. (1984). Is the ileo-caecal Peyer's patch in ruminants a mammalian "bursa-equivalent"? Acta Pathol Microbiol Immunol Scand A *92*, 77-79.

Miyazawa, K., Aso, H., Kanaya, T., Kido, T., Minashima, T., Watanabe, K., Ohwada, S., Kitazawa, H., Rose, M.T., Tahara, K., *et al.* (2006). Apoptotic process of porcine intestinal M cells. Cell Tissue Res *323*, 425-432.

Miyazawa, K., Kanaya, T., Takakura, I., Tanaka, S., Hondo, T., Watanabe, H., Rose, M.T., Kitazawa, H., Yamaguchi, T., Katamine, S., *et al.* (2010). Transcytosis of murine-adapted bovine spongiform encephalopathy agents in an in vitro bovine M cell model. J Virol *84*, 12285-12291.

Moll, R., Franke, W.W., Schiller, D.L., Geiger, B., and Krepler, R. (1982). The catalog of human cytokeratins: patterns of expression in normal epithelia, tumors and cultured cells. Cell *31*, 11-24.

Neutra, M.R., Frey, A., and Kraehenbuhl, J.P. (1996). Epithelial M cells: gateways for mucosal infection and immunization. Cell *86*, 345-348.

Neutra, M.R., Mantis, N.J., and Kraehenbuhl, J.P. (2001). Collaboration of epithelial cells with organized mucosal lymphoid tissues. Nat Immunol *2*, 1004-1009.

Rautenberg, K., Cichon, C., Heyer, G., Demel, M., and Schmidt, M.A. (1996). Immunocytochemical characterization of the follicle-associated epithelium of Peyer's patches: anti-cytokeratin 8 antibody (clone 4.1.18) as a molecular marker for rat M cells. Eur J Cell Biol *71*, 363-370.

Reynolds, J.D., and Morris, B. (1983). The evolution and involution of Peyer's patches in fetal and postnatal sheep. Eur J Immunol *13*, 627-635.

Savidge, T.C., Smith, M.W., James, P.S., and Aldred, P. (1991). Salmonella-induced M-cell formation in germ-free mouse Peyer's patch tissue. Am J Pathol *139*, 177-184.

Sierro, F., Pringault, E., Assman, P.S., Kraehenbuhl, J.P., and Debard, N. (2000). Transient expression of M-cell phenotype by enterocyte-like cells of the follicle-associated epithelium of mouse Peyer's patches. Gastroenterology *119*, 734-743.

Takakura, I., Miyazawa, K., Kanaya, T., Itani, W., Watanabe, K., Ohwada, S., Watanabe, H., Hondo, T., Rose, M.T., Mori, T., *et al.* (2011). Orally administered prion protein is incorporated by m cells and spreads into lymphoid tissues with macrophages in prion protein knockout mice. Am J Pathol *179*, 1301-1309.

Zhou, Q., Toivola, D.M., Feng, N., Greenberg, H.B., Franke, W.W., and Omary, M.B. (2003). Keratin 20 helps maintain intermediate filament organization in intestinal epithelia. Mol Bio

2

Cytokeratins of the Liver and Intestine Epithelial Cells During Development and Disease

Priti Chougule and Suchitra Sumitran-Holgersson
Sahlgrenska Academy, University of Gothenburg
Sweden

1. Introduction

A large part of the cytoplasm of the cells consists of components forming cytoskeleton. The constituents of the cytoskeleton in epithelial cells are actin-containing microfilaments, tubulin-containing microtubules and intermediate size filaments. The intermediate filaments are called as cytokeratins (CK). Thus, cytokeratins are a family of many different filament-forming proteins (polypeptides) with specific physicochemical properties and are normal components of epithelial cell cytoskeleton. CK are expressed in various types of epithelia in different combinations. Cytokeratins account for about 80% of the total protein content in differentiated cells of stratified epithelia (Pekny and Lane 2007). In both human and murine stratified epidermis, CK account for 25–35% of the extracted proteins(Bowden, Quinlan et al. 1984). The expression of proteins forming intermediate filaments can change when epithelial cells develop into mesenchymal cells and vice versa(Moll, Moll et al. 1984). For example, during neural tube formation, CK-producing ectodermal cells change into vimentin-producing mesenchymal cells, whereas during the formation of renal tubules vimentin-producing mesenchymal cells change into CK-producing epithelial cells(Moll, et al. 1984). Different types of cytokeratins are distinguished according to various characteristics, such as physicochemical properties, or according to the cells and tissues that produce certain CK. In simple, non-stratified epithelia these proteins are different than those in stratified epithelia. Epithelial cells in simple as well as in stratified epithelia always synthesize particular CK on a regular basis. These cytokeratins are referred to as the primary keratins of epithelial cells, such as CK8/CK18 in simple epithelia (Pekny and Lane 2007) or CK5/CK14 in stratified(Moll, Franke et al. 1982). In addition or instead, these epithelial cells can also produce secondary CK, such as CK7/CK19 in simple epithelia or CK15 and CK6/CK16 in stratified epithelia.

During embryonic development of simple to stratified epithelia, different cytokeratins are expressed (Banksschlegel 1982). Cells of the single-layered precursor of the human epidermis produce the same types of CK that are characteristic of simple epithelia, namely CK8, CK18 and CK19 (Dale, Holbrook et al. 1985). With the onset of stratification, different cytokeratins are expressed in the basal and suprabasal layers, e.g. CK5 is produced instead of CK8. With the onset of keratinization, CK1 and CK10 are added to the cytoskeleton in the suprabasal cell layers. Around the same time, there is a change in the expression of certain keratin genes, with large keratins being produced with the onset of keratinization, and smaller ones no longer being synthesized (Banksschlegel 1982).

In medical diagnosis, antibodies against various cytokeratins have been used to characterize a wide variety of epithelial tumors. For example immunohistochemical detection of cytokeratin can identify micrometastases, not detected by conventional hematoxylin and eosin staining, Also serum cytokeratins levels are widely used as markers of tumors of epithelial origin (Linder 2007).

2. Role of keratins

The main function of cytokeratins is to give mechanical strength to the epithelial cells. But importance of this function depends upon the cell type. The epithelial layer which is constantly exposed to mechanical stress like epidermis, this function is important but this function is not so much important in single layered epithelial cells of internal organs which are not exposed to much mechanical stress. In polarized epithelial cells like intestinal epithelial cells, keratins play the role to maintain the cell polarity (Owens and Lane 2003; Oriolo, Wald et al. 2007). CK are not evenly distributed throughout the cytoplasm. CK19 is most abundant at the apical end below microvilli. Defect in CK19 expression affects the polarity of the cell (Salas, Rodriguez et al. 1997). In rat intestine, staining of CK8 and CK21 is observed at the cell periphery of absorptive cells while staining of CK19 is observed at the central region (Habtezion, Toivola et al. 2011). Cytokeratin filaments are also important in intercellular context. They are attached to the desmosomes as well as hemi-desmosomes. Thus they help in cell-cell adhesion and also attachment of the epithelial cells with the underlining connective tissue. Besides this structural function CK also plays a role in transport of some membrane proteins (Coulombe, Tong et al. 2004; Zhou, Cadrin et al. 2006; Kim and Coulombe 2007). In CK8 null mice, it is observed that there is abnormality in the distribution of apical surface markers. Regional differences in the expression of syntaxin-3, intestinal alkaline phosphatase and CFTR chloride channel proteins were observed in small intestine of CK8 null animals (Oshima 2002). Role of keratins in cell signaling is also proposed. Simple epithelial keratin pair; CK8/CK18 interact with Fas and TNF-alpha receptors (Caulin, Ware et al. 2000; Oshima 2002; Paramio and Jorcano 2002). Cells deficient in CK8 and CK18 are more sensitive to TNF induced cell death (Inada, Izawa et al. 2001).

Role of CK in apoptosis is documented in many studies (Ku, Liao et al. 1997; Oshima 2002; Owens and Lane 2003). In apoptosis process, the pre-apoptotic event is the hyper phosphorylation of keratin filament. These CK are then degraded by caspase. Only type I CK are susceptible to caspase mediated proteolysis and not type II CK. Phosphorylated CK8/CK18 pair is the substrate for pro-caspase 3 and 9 (Lee, Schickling et al. 2002; Dinsdale, Lee et al. 2004). Breakdown of this keratin pair results in the collapse of cytoplasmic and nuclear cytoskeleton which leads to the condensation of chromatin, which is the hallmark of apoptosis process. Organized cell fragmentation during apoptosis is essential to prevent the induction of inflammatory response. Programmed destruction of CK network is essential for this. Defect in CK composition may affect the sensitivity of the cell to apoptosis which is proposed in case of colonic hyperplasia. But there are also some studies in which (Ku and Omary 2000) it is stated that hyperphosphorylation of CK does not make the cells susceptible to apoptosis. It only affects the dimer formation (Strnad, Windoffer et al. 2001).

At this point in time, the expression of cytokeratins during development of human liver and intestine need clarification and the functional importance of these proteins in liver and intestine diseases require updating. Furthermore, much is known now about the expression, assembly, and function of CK in keratinized epithelial cells, the main features being the tight coupling between CK pair switch and cell terminal differentiation (protection barrier) and the vital role of CK intermediate filaments in cell mechanical integrity. However, the picture about non-keratinizing epithelia, like the hepatic tissue, remains quite unclear. In this review we will address these issues and also highlight the role of CK in liver and intestinal diseases.

3. Cytokeratin expression during liver development and regeneration

During embryological development, around 8 gestational weeks (GW), bipotential hepatoblasts stream from the hepatic diverticulum, and differentiate into both hepatocytes and ductal plate cells. Human intrahepatic biliary system arises from the ductal plate, which is a double-layered cylindrical structure located at the interface between portal mesenchyme and primitive hepatocytes. Around 12 GW, the ductal plate gradually undergoes remodeling; some parts of the ductal plate disappear and other parts migrate into the portal mesenchyme. Around 20 GW, the migrated duct cells transform into immature bile ducts and peribiliary glands (Bateman and Hubscher 2010). Around postnatal 3 months, some immature peribiliary glands transform into pancreatic acinar cells. These embryological progenitor cells express a broad range of cytokeratins - CK8, CK18, CK19 and (transiently) CK14. Ductal plate cells continue to express CK8, CK18 and CK19 and at 20 weeks of gestation begin to express CK7. This immunophenotype is retained by mature bile ducts at birth. Developing hepatocytes express CK8 and CK18 but not CK7 or CK19 (Desmet, Vaneyken et al. 1990).

It is now believed that the role of progenitor cells in liver regeneration may have similarities to embryological liver development. Studies have attempted to define the nature and position of progenitor cells within the liver in a variety of ways. This has included study of animal models of liver diseases, embryological human livers in cell culture and *in vivo* (Nava, Westgren et al. 2005) (Nowak et al. 2005) and adult human livers in cell culture (Herrera, Bruno et al. 2006) (Khuu, Najimi et al. 2007) and *in vivo* (Chatzipantelis, Lazaris et al. 2006). In our own studies we demonstrated that *in vitro* expanded human fetal liver progenitor cells express CK18, CK8 and some CK19 (Figure 1). In fact, these double positive (positive for CK18 and CK19) later differentiate into cells expressing either only CK18 (hepatocytes) or only CK19 (bile duct cells-cholangiocytes). Interestingly, a cell type termed the 'oval' cell has been described as a putative hepatic stem cell in animal (especially rat) models. These cells appear in the portal and periportal regions of animal livers within a few days of liver injury and may express biliary markers such as CK7 and CK19 as well as hepatocyte markers such as pyruvate kinase isoenzyme L-PK, albumin and alpha-fetoprotein (AFP). They may also express other markers such as OV-6, an antibody raised in mice and recognizing epitopes within CK14 and CK19 in rats (Vessey and Hall 2001). Oval cells differentiate into hepatocytes via 'transitional' hepatocytes.

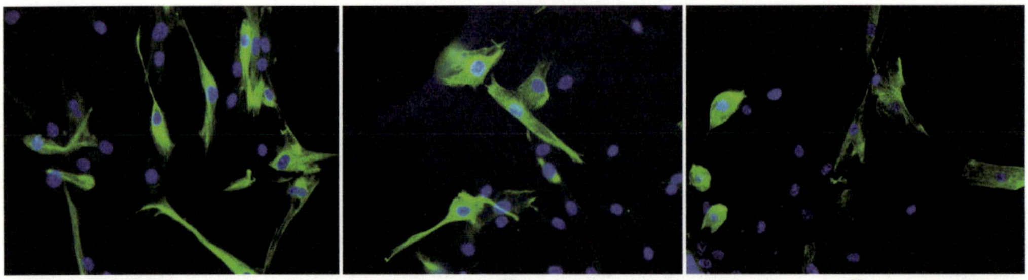

A B C

Fig. 1. Immunofluorescence staining of in vitro expanded human fetal liver progenitor cells showing expression of (A) CK18 in almost all cells, while (B) CK8 and (C) CK19 expression was found only in some cells.

4. Distribution of cytoskeleton intermediate filaments during fetal hepatocyte differentiation

During fetal development, the construction of the liver parenchyma depends on the intricate relationship of intercellular contacts between epithelial cells and between epithelial and mesenchymal cells. In the early stages of fetal rat (Vassy, Rigaut et al. 1990) and human (Nava, Westgren et al. 2005) development, the liver is mainly a hematopoietic organ and hepatocytes represent fewer than 40% of all liver cells. In rats, at this time, cytokeratin filaments are scarce but are uniformly distributed inside the cytoplasm (Vassy, Irinopoulou et al. 1997). A coexpression of desmin and cytokeratin is found in some cells. Intercellular contacts between epithelial and mesenchymal cells are more numerous than between epithelial cells. Later in development, contacts between hepatocytes become more numerous and bile canaliculi become well developed. The density of cytokeratin filaments increases and appears to be very high near the bile canaliculi. In adult liver, hepatocytes are arranged in a "muralium simplex" architecture (one-cell-thick sheets) (Elias and Scherrick, 1969). Cytokeratin filaments show a symmetrical distribution in relation to the nuclear region. The highest density of filaments is found near the cytoplasmic membrane (Vassy et al. 1996). During development of fetal hepatocytes variations in cytokeratin networks can be correlated with different steps in cell differentiation. The special expression of intermediate filament proteins in fetal liver cells is reflective of the particular environment of the fetal liver in terms of extracellular matrix composition and intercellular contacts. Furthermore, the intracellular distribution of these CK proteins could be influenced by the cellular environment.

Immunohistochemistry can help to identify the various components of the intrahepatic biliary system in normal liver tissue. Markers such as polyclonal carcinoembryonic antigen and CD10 are also quite widely used in diagnostic practice to highlight bile canalicular differentiation in hepatocellular neoplasms and clearly identify the same structures within normal liver. CK7 and CK19 are strongly expressed by interlobular bile ducts, intraportal and intralobular bile ductules and the biliary epithelial cells that partly line the canals of Herring (Bateman and Hubscher 2010). It has been suggested that the individual CK7+ and CK19+ cells that partly line the canals of Herring represent hepatic progenitor cells. Biliary epithelial cells also express CK8 and CK18. In contrast, normal hepatocytes express CK8 and CK18 but not CK7 or CK19.

Thus, the liver forms a multicellular system, where parenchymal cells (i.e., hepatocytes) exert diverse metabolic functions and nonparenchymal epithelial cells (e.g., biliary epithelial cells) usually serve structural and other accessory purposes. In terms of differential CK gene expression, the data accumulated so far demonstrates that parenchymal cells can contain as few as one single CK pair, whereas nonparenchymal cells contain more than two CKs, one of them being a representative of those found in epidermis. Moreover, the distribution of the CK IF networks present in the different cell types varies a lot and can often be linked to the cell specialization. However, the function(s) played by these IF proteins in this multicellular tissue remains a major issue.

5. Role of cytokeratins in liver diseases

The concept of progenitor cells with the ability for maturation into biliary epithelium and hepatocytes is supported by *in vivo* studies of human liver disease. For example, CK7 immunohistochemistry in chronic viral hepatitis and autoimmune hepatitis highlights a bile ductular reaction and individual cells within hepatic lobules thought to represent progenitor cells. CK7 expression is also seen in hepatocytes in these conditions. This has been interpreted as *in vivo* evidence that progenitor cells can differentiate into ductular cells and mature hepatocytes in response to the chronic liver injury associated with these diseases, in contrast to the previously held view that mature hepatocytes at the limiting plate transform via metaplasia into biliary ductal cells. The degree of bile ductular reaction, progenitor cell numbers and proportion of hepatocytes expressing CK7 increases in parallel with disease grade (activity) and stage (Eleazar, Memeo et al. 2004; Fotiadu, Tzioufa et al. 2004). The positive association between hepatocyte CK7 expression and disease stage suggests that the increased extracellular matrix present in severe fibrosis and cirrhosis may produce a survival or maturation factor for progenitor cells (Eleazar, Memeo et al. 2004).

Mutations in the genes encoding CK proteins either directly cause or predispose their carriers to many human diseases (Coulombe and Omary 2002; Omary, Coulombe et al. 2004). The liver appears to be the primary target organ, with mutations in the genes KRT8, KRT18 and KRT19, which encode CK8, CK18 and CK19, respectively. Such mutations have been reported to predispose individuals to liver diseases (Ku, Wright et al. 1997; Ku, Gish et al. 2001). Furthermore, CK also have disease relevance in other contexts e.g they are important in the formation of hepatocyte Mallory-Denk bodies, which are hepatic inclusions observed in various chronic liver diseases (Zatloukal, French et al. 2007). Mallory-Denk bodies are found mainly in hepatocytes of patients with alcoholic and nonalcoholic steatohepatitis, but are also found in the hepatocytes of patients with primary biliary cirrhosis, hepatocellular carcinomas, and copper metabolism disorders (Zatloukal, French et al. 2007). Stress conditions may affect not only CK expression profiles, but also the levels of CK expression and posttranslational modification. For example, increased CK phophorylation is a marker of tissue injury and disease progression in human and mouse liver (Omary, Ku et al. 2009). Under certain stress conditions, increased CK expression may contribute to important cytoprotection provided by CK8 and CK18 in the liver. However, the importance of such upregulation has not been directly demonstrated (Ku, Strnad et al. 2007). These findings are supported by the observation of CK8 and CK18 over expression after injury in patients with primary biliary cirrhosis (Fickert, Trauner et al. 2003). In our own studies, we have found markedly increased levels of CK19 expression in patients with autoimmune liver diseases such as primary sclerosing cholangitis, primary biliary cirrhosis and autoimmune hepatitis (Figure 2). We currently do not know the significance of increased CK19 expression in these diseases, but speculate that it may be a marker of liver tissue injury or disease progression in PSC and PBC patients.

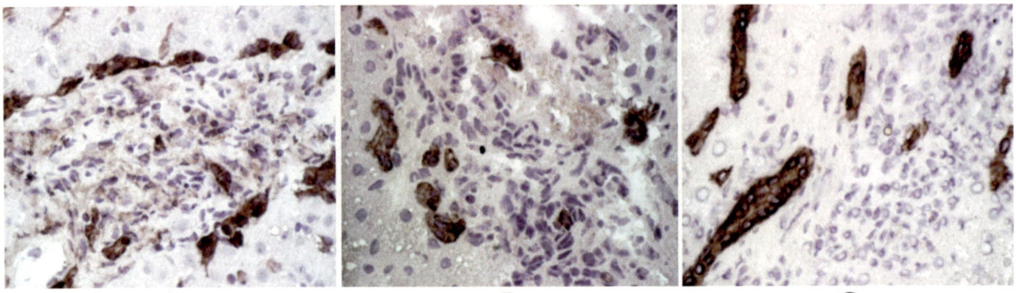

A B C

Fig. 2. Immunohistochemical staining of liver biopsies from patients with (A) Primary sclerosing cholangitis, (B) Primary biliary cirrhosis and (C) Autoimmune hepatitis showing markedly increased expression of CK19 in the bile ducts of these patients.

6. Understanding CK-related liver diseases via transgenic animal models

Important information regarding keratin function *in vivo* has been obtained by the use of CK knockout and transgenic mice which has lead to the identification of human diseases that are related to mutations in genes encoding CK (Ku, Strnad et al. 2007). CK8-deficient C57BL/6 mice were the first mice to be generated. These mice exhibited liver hemorrhage and greater than 90% embryo lethality (Baribault, Price et al. 1993). When the surviving mice were further backcrossed onto an FVB background, it resulted in generation of mice with 50% embryo lethality. Although the surviving mice had a normal life span, they exhibited an ulcerative colitis–like phenotype (Baribault, Penner et al. 1994; Toivola, Krishnan et al. 2004; Habtezion, Toivola et al. 2005) and considerable hepatocyte fragility and susceptibility to liver injury (Loranger, Duclos et al. 1997). Although both CK8- and CK18-deficient mice lack hepatocyte keratin filaments, their phenotype is partially different. For example, no embryo lethality or colitis is observed in CK18-deficient mixed-background mice because of functional redundancy with CK19 (Magin, Schroder et al. 1998). However, both CK8-null and CK18-null mice have increased hepatocyte fragility (Loranger, Duclos et al. 1997; Ku and Omary 2006) and susceptibility to hepatocyte apoptosis (Oshima 2002; Marceau, Schutte et al. 2007). The first clear and detailed link between CK and liver disease came from mice that over expressed the R90C mutant of CK18. These mice exhibited mild chronic hepatitis and substantial hepatocyte fragility upon liver perfusion (Ku, Michie et al. 1995), with dramatic susceptibility to liver injury (Ku, Michie et al. 1996). It was this observation that led to the testing and initial identification of mutations in KRT18 and then KRT8 (Ku, Strnad et al. 2007) in patients with liver disease.

Transgenic mouse studies have also helped undersand how naturally occurring human mutations in the genes encoding CK predispose to liver disease. For example, over expression of the natural human G62C K8 mutant in transgenic mice leads to increased hepatocyte apoptosis and liver injury (Ku and Omary 2006). This predisposition is related to a mutation-mediated conformational change that blocks CK8 S74 phosphorylation by stress kinases (Ku and Omary 2006; Tao, Nakamichi et al. 2006). The importance of CK phosphorylation in protecting cells from stress is further supported by the increased risk for liver injury in mice that over express the S53A K18 phosphomutant (Ku, Michie et al. 1998). Furthermore, transgenic mice that over express the S34A K18 mutant, cannot bind 14-3-3 proteins, leading to limited mitotic arrest (Ku, Michie et al. 2002). Altogether, these genetically engineered mice ultimately led to the association of keratin mutations with human liver disease and to understanding some of the involved pathogenic mechanisms.

7. CK as serum markers and CK variants in liver diseases

Mutations in the genes encoding keratins cause several human diseases, (Coulombe and Omary 2002; Omary, Coulombe et al. 2004). The association of CK variants with human acute and chronic liver disease is supported by numerous studies. For chronic liver disease, KRT8 and KRT18 variants are found to be overrepresented in patients with end stage liver disease of multiple etiologies (Zatloukal, French et al. 2007). Interestingly, PBC was the first human disease reported to be associated with CK19 and CK8 variants (Zhong, Strnad et al. 2009).

CK or CK fragments circulating in serum, which are released from apoptotic or necrotic tumor and non-tumor cells, have been used as tumor markers for monitoring disease progression in several cancers (Linder 2007). The most commonly used markers are tissue polypeptide antigen (TPA; a mixture of CK8, CK18, and CK19), tissue polypeptide–specific antigen (TPS; derived from CK18), cytokeratin fragment 21-1 (CYFRA 21-1; derived from CK19) (Leers, Kolgen et al. 1999; Marceau, Schutte et al. 2007). High TPS levels have been reported in several liver disorders (Gonzalez-Quintela, Mallo et al. 2006).

8. Autoantibodies specific for CK in human liver diseases

Autoantibodies specific for CK have been reported in autoimmune and malignant liver diseases. A sub fraction of autoimmune hepatitis (AIH) patients harbors high titers of antibodies specific for CK8, CK18, and CK19 that decrease after steroid treatment (Murota, Nishioka et al. 2001). Moreover, CK8- and CK18-specific antibodies have been detected in patients with de novo AIH after liver transplantation, whereas liver transplant recipients without de novo AIH were seronegative for these antibodies (Inui, Sogo et al. 2005). These antibodies may develop as a consequence of recurrent or chronic cell death, which leads to exposure of the immune system to cytoplasmic proteins that are not normally present in the circulation. Other CK-targeted autoantibodies include antibodies specific for CK8/CK18; these have been found in association with cryptogenic acute liver failure, which may suggest an autoimmune pathogenesis (Berna, Ma et al. 2007). Proteomic analysis has revealed an increased frequency of CK8-specific antibodies in patients with hepatocellular carcinoma compared with patients with chronic viral hepatitis. However, controversy exists regarding these results (Le Naour, Brichory et al. 2002; Li, Chen et al. 2008). Similar to the situation of CK serum markers, the presence of CK-specific autoantibodies may provide potentially useful clinical tools for diagnosis and determining prognosis and treatment response, but additional studies are required.

9. Intestinal cytokeratins – Model to study cytokeratin changes during differentiation and apoptosis

Main function of cytokeratins is to give mechanical support to the cell. But along with this static function they also play a role in dynamic processes like mitosis, cell movement and differentiation (Chandler, Calnek et al. 1991; Corden and McLean 1996; Ku, Zhou et al. 1999). Cytokeratin composition of the cell changes during these processes fulfilling the different needs of the cell during these processes, e.g. in non-dividing terminally differentiated cells, the role of the CK is to give a physical support to the cell which role is not so much important in rapidly dividing cells where rapid CK remodeling is essential. During proliferation phase it is important to respond rapidly to the cell signals by undergoing polymerization and depolymarization. As CK heterodimers differ in their viscoelastic properties and ability to undergo rapid polymerazation-demolymerization, CK pattern also changes in the same epithelial cell during division phase and maturation phase.

Intestinal epithelial cells provide an excellent model, for the study of these diverse functions, as these cells undergo proliferation, differentiation and apoptosis processes within a very short period of time. During their migration from crypt to villus region, cells undergo division cycles in the crypt region, differentiation phase along the villus and apoptosis at the tip of the villi. All these phases are thus temporally arranged along the crypt-villus axis. By studying CK pattern along crypt-villus axis, we can speculate how CK pattern changes during different phases of the cells.

In intestinal epithelial cells major type II cytokeratin present is CK8 (Moll, Franke et al. 1982; Zhou, Toivola et al. 2003; Omary, Ku et al. 2009; Habtezion, Toivola et al. 2011). Presence of CK7 is reported in some studies (Moll, Franke et al. 1982; Casanova, Bravo et al. 1995; Wildi, Kleeff et al. 1999; Zhou, Toivola et al. 2003; Schutte, Henfling et al. 2004; Toivola, Krishnan et al. 2004; Moll, Divo et al. 2008; Omary, Ku et al. 2009; Habtezion, Toivola et al. 2011) while there are also some reports stating the absence of this CK in the intestine (Ramaekers, Huysmans et al. 1987; Oriolo, Wald et al. 2007). Several type I cytokeratins are present in intestinal epithelial cells. Along with usual partner of CK8, i.e. CK18, these cells also contains CK19 and CK20. Presence of multiple type I cytokeratins is not redundant as gene replacement studies have shown that defect in any type I cytokeratin may lead to defect in the cells morphology and function. Additional cytokeratin filaments present in the intestine may be due to requirement of more structural strength by these cells as among the internal organs, intestine is subjected to more mechanical stress because of the movement of the luminal content (Owens, Wilson et al. 2004).

10. Expression along crypt-villus axis

The intestinal cells along the crypt-villus axis differ in structure as well as in function which in also reflected in different cytokeratins composition of these cells (Quaroni, Calnek et al. 1991). These changes along the crypt-villus axis are more apparent in animals than in human intestine. CK8, CK18 and C19 were found to be present along entire crypt-villus axis in humans while in rats CK18 is absent in villus cells. In rats, crypt cells also showed presence of CK7 (Omary, Ku et al. 2009). Human CK20 and its rat homologous CK21 is present exclusively in differentiated villus cells (Zhou, Toivola et al. 2003). Till today it has been found to be difficult to attribute a specific function to individual keratin so it is difficult to predict the reason for these differences. One hypothesis is that cytokeratin filaments are observed to be associated with both desmosomes as well as microvillar rootlets. These components are present only in mature villus cells and not in immature crypt cells (Fath, Obenauf et al. 1990; Heintzelman and Mooseker 1990; Quaroni 1999). And also the extensive cytokeratin filaments are necessary to maintain the structural strength in mature villus cells, while it is deleterious for rapidly dividing crypt cells. CK20 expression in villus enterocyte may be related to the differentiated state of these cells and also the apoptosis process observed in the villus tip cells, as CK20 plays role in changes in cell shape required for exfoliation (Zhou, Cadrin et al. 2006). CK19 is preferentially localized in the apical domain of the several polarized cultured cells and down regulation of this cytokeratin using antisense nucleotides decreased the number of microvilli and also mis-sorted the targeting of apically distributed proteins. Distribution of basolateral proteins remains unaffected. But it is difficult to attribute these changes to the CK19, as changes in microtubules and microfilament was also observed in these cells. Thus, both crypt and villus cells different in the structure and function which can be observed in their different cytokeratin composition.

11. Cytokeratin changes during fetal development

Cytokeratin composition of the cells varies during embryonic development as well (Quaroni, Calnek et al. 1991). Changes in CK composition during fetal intestinal development were studied in rats. These changes are similar to the changes observed during differentiation in adult mucosa. In these animals stratified epithelium is present at the 15-16 days of gestation during which time CK19 is predominantly present with small amount of CK8. Expression of CK21 was observed when brush border and apical cytoplasmic terminal web formation starts at 18-19 days of gestation. In humans K20 appears at embryonic week 8 (Moll, Divo et al. 2008). There is also increase in the relative abundance of CK8 at this period. In adult human intestine expression of CK20 is observed along the villus cells while in fetal intestine some CK20 - negative cells were observed. Such mosaic distribution of CK20 - negative cells was not observed in fetal rat intestine (Moll, Zimbelmann et al. 1993).

12. Cytokeratin changes in animal and human intestine

A difference is observed in CK composition between rat and human intestinal epithelial cells. In rats, CK8 and CK19 are the major keratins, while CK18 and CK21 are less abundant. CK21 is homologous to human CK20 (Calnek and Quaroni 1993; Bragulla and Homberger 2009). This keratin is present only in differentiated villus cells in both rats and human. In rats, only type I keratin, CK19 is present in crypt cells while in humans CK18 and CK19 were found to be present in these cells. Uniform distribution of CK8, CK18 and CK19 has been observed along the crypt villus axis in humans while in rats, the common partner of CK8 i.e. CK18 was not observed in villus cells.

We studied the keratin expression in normal adult intestinal sample and also in cultured epithelial cells from these samples (n=5). Fig. 3 (a-d) shows cytokeratin filament network of human small intestine stained for CK8, CK18, CK19 and CK20 respectively. Entire epithelial layer showed positive staining for CK8, CK18 and CK19. But staining intensity for these CK is less in crypt cells compared to the intensity in villus cells. Bright CK positive staining is observed near the apical and basolateral membrane along with cytoplasmic staining for CK8, CK18 and CK19 but not for CK20.

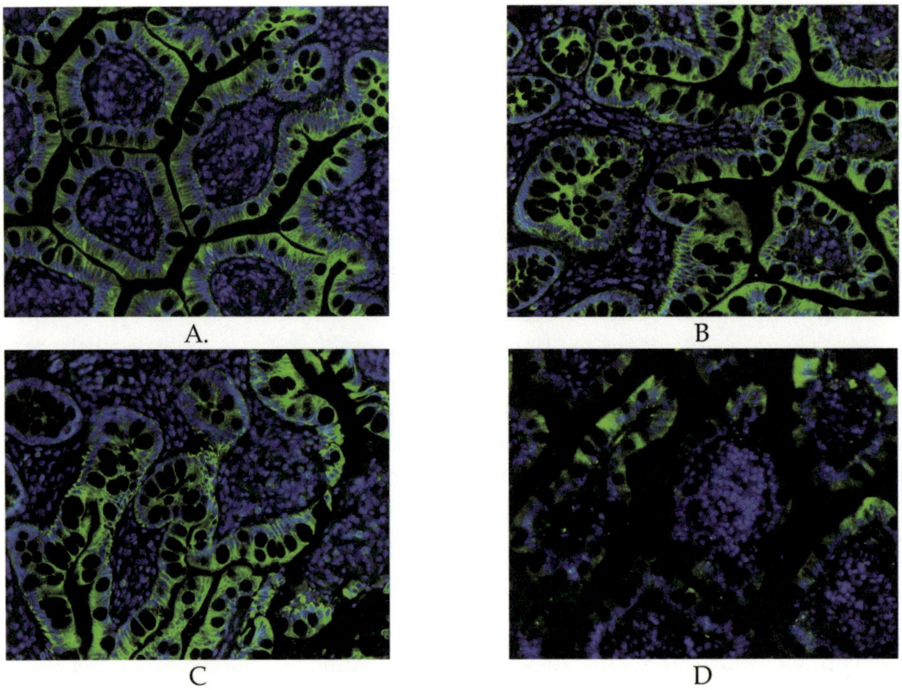

Fig. 3. Human small intestine stained for cytokeratins. Positive immunofluorescence staining for (A) CK8, (B) CK18, (C) CK19 and (D) CK20 was observed. These cells showed positive staining in the cytoplasm but intense staining is also observed along the membrane for CK8, CK18 and CK19.

13. Cytokeratin and related diseases

Cytokeratin mutation and intestinal disorders is the subject of many studies (Owens and Lane 2004; Owens, Wilson et al. 2004). As CK8 is the only Type II cytokeratin present in the intestine, mutation in CK8 affect the intestinal epithelium. Intestinal phenotype of CK8 null mice is similar to IBD phenotype. There are studies reporting the mutation in CK genes in subset of IBD patients (Owens, Wilson et al. 2004). A single amino acid change in CK8 leads to homo-dimer formation (Owens, Wilson et al. 2004) and CK are rapidly degraded when are not present as a heterodimer. This impaired CK assembly may make these cells more prone to the mechanical damage and creating a defect in the integrity of epithelial layer. And it is also observed that CK defect may affect the permeability of intestinal epithelial layer (Owens, Wilson et al. 2004; Toivola, Krishnan et al. 2004) which is one of the features observed in IBD patients. Apical membrane proteins of intestinal epithelial cells can affect the micro-flora present in the lumen (Hooper, Falk et al. 2000). Cytokeratin defects can alter the membrane proteins and hence the luminal flora which may result into the inflammatory reactions (Ameen, Figueroa et al. 2001). Thus type II cytokeratin mutation may contribute to a risk of IBD. Mutation in CK18 does not adversely affect the intestine probably because of the presence of other type I cytokeratins (Zhou, Toivola et al. 2003; Hesse, Grund et al. 2007). Even though cytokeratin related diseases are rare, many studies revealed that mutations in these proteins, predisposes the cell to diseases.

Tissue	CK7	CK8	CK18	CK19	CK20	Ref.
LIVER						
Developing hepatocytes	+	+	+	+	-	(Omary, Coulombe et al. 2004; Bateman and Hubscher 2010)
Developing bile ducts	(+)	+	+	+	-	(Bateman and Hubscher 2010)
Adult Hepatocytes	-	+	+	-	-	(Omary, Coulombe et al. 2004; Bateman and Hubscher 2010)
Adult bile ducts	+	-	-	+	-	(Bateman and Hubscher 2010)
Liver diseases						
Primary biliary cirrhosis	+	+	+	+	-	(Fickert, Trauner et al. 2003; Bateman and Hubscher 2010)
Autoimmune hepatitis	(+)	-	-	-	+	(Bateman and Hubscher 2010)
Primary Sclerosing Cholangitis	+	-	-	+	-	(Bateman and Hubscher 2010)
Alcoholic cirrhosis	+	-	-	(+)	-	(Vaneyken, Sciot et al. 1988; Ku, Strnad et al. 2007)
Hepatocellularcarcinoma	(-)	+	+	(?)	-	(Chu and Weiss 2002; Tot 2002; Moll, Divo et al. 2008)
Cholangiocarcinoma	+	+	+	-	-	(Chu and Weiss 2002; Tot 2002; Moll, Divo et al. 2008)
Intestine						
Rodent crypt cells	+	(+)	+	+	-	(Flint, Pemberton et al. 1994; Zhou, Toivola et al. 2003)
Rodent villus cells	-	+	-	+	+	(Quaroni, Calnek et al. 1991; Flint, Pemberton et al. 1994)
Human crypt cells	+ (?)	+	+	+	-	(Owens, Wilson et al. 2004; Toivola, Krishnan et al. 2004)
Human villus cells	+ (?)	+	+	+	+	(Owens, Wilson et al. 2004; Toivola, Krishnan et al. 2004)

Intestine diseases						
Colon cancer	+ (some cases)	+	+	+	+	(Harbaum, Pollheimer et al. 2011; Karantza 2011)
IBD	NR	-	NR	NR	NR	(Caulin, Ware et al. 2000; Owens and Lane 2004)
Colonic hyperplasia	NR	-	NR	NR	NR	(Baribault, Penner et al. 1994)

Table 1. Cytokeratin expression in Livers and intestine

14. Conclusion

The study of CK expression in the liver and intestine during development provides a useful insight into the mechanisms underlying stem cell activity and tissue remodeling in embryology. The previous concept that mature hepatocytes undergo metaplasia into bile ductular cells is now questioned and a new hypothesis that bipotential progenitor cells residing in the canals of herring may play a more important role in understanding the mechanisms of various liver diseases where cytokeratin expression has been found to aid in clinical diagnosis. Individuals with mutations in the genes encoding CK are more susceptible to various liver and intestinal diseases. However, further studies which include specific acute and chronic liver and intestinal disorders are required to fully assess the relative importance of CK mutations. Furthermore CK expression in intestinal epithelia is very complex and restricted to specific enterocyte subpopulations, yet the functional implications are not known. Further work in understanding the functions of CK7, CK19 and CK20 in the intestine is validated. Thus, the complex but interesting field of cytokeratins provides an important area for further investigation.

15. References

Ameen, N. A., Y. Figueroa, et al. (2001). "Anomalous apical plasma membrane phenotype in CK8-deficient mice indicates a novel role for intermediate filaments in the polarization of simple epithelia." *Journal of Cell Science* 114(3): 563-575.

Banksschlegel, S. P. (1982). "Keratin Alterations during Embryonic Epidermal Differentiation - a Presage of Adult Epidermal Maturation." *Journal of Cell Biology* 93(3): 551-559.

Baribault, H., J. Penner, et al. (1994). "Colorectal Hyperplasia and Inflammation in Keratin 8-Deficient Evb/N Mice." *Genes & Development* 8(24): 2964-2973.

Baribault, H., J. Price, et al. (1993). "Midgestational Lethality in Mice Lacking Keratin-8." *Genes & Development* 7(7A): 1191-1202.

Bateman, A. C. and S. G. Hubscher (2010). "Cytokeratin expression as an aid to diagnosis in medical liver biopsies." *Histopathology* 56(4): 415-425.

Berna, W., Y. Ma, et al. (2007). "The significance of autoantibodies and immunoglobulins in acute liver failure: A cohort study." *Journal of Hepatology* 47(5): 664-670.

Bowden, P. E., R. A. Quinlan, et al. (1984). "Proteolytic Modification of Acidic and Basic Keratins during Terminal Differentiation of Mouse and Human-Epidermis." *European Journal of Biochemistry* 142(1): 29-36.

Bragulla, H. H. and D. G. Homberger (2009). "Structure and functions of keratin proteins in simple, stratified, keratinized and cornified epithelia." *Journal of Anatomy* 214(4): 516-559.

Calnek, D. and A. Quaroni (1993). "Differential Localization by Insitu Hybridization of Distinct Keratin Messenger-Rna Species during Intestinal Epithelial-Cell Development and Differentiation." *Differentiation* 53(2): 95-104.

Casanova, L., A. Bravo, et al. (1995). "Tissue-Specific and Efficient Expression of the Human Simple Epithelial Keratin-8 Gene in Transgenic Mice." *Journal of Cell Science* 108: 811-820.

Caulin, C., C. F. Ware, et al. (2000). "Keratin-dependent, epithelial resistance to tumor necrosis factor-induced apoptosis." *Journal of Cell Biology* 149(1): 17-22.

Chandler, J. S., D. Calnek, et al. (1991). "Identification and Characterization of Rat Intestinal Keratins - Molecular-Cloning of Cdnas Encoding Cytokeratin-8, Cytokeratin-19, and a New 49-Kda Type-I Cytokeratin (Cytokeratin-21) Expressed by Differentiated Intestinal Epithelial-Cells." *Journal of Biological Chemistry* 266(18): 11932-11938.

Chatzipantelis, P., A. C. Lazaris, et al. (2006). "Cytokeratin-7, cytokeratin-19, and c-Kit: Immunoreaction during the evolution stages of primary biliary cirrhosis." *Hepatology Research* 36(3): 182-187.

Chu, P. G. and L. M. Weiss (2002). "Keratin expression in human tissues and neoplasms." *Histopathology* 40(5): 403-439.

Corden, L. D. and W. H. McLean (1996). "Human keratin diseases: hereditary fragility of specific epithelial tissues." *Experimental Dermatology* 5(6): 297-307.

Coulombe, P. A. and M. B. Omary (2002). "'Hard' and 'soft' principles defining the structure, function and regulation of keratin intermediate filaments." *Current Opinion in Cell Biology* 14(1): 110-122.

Coulombe, P. A., X. M. Tong, et al. (2004). "Great promises yet to be fulfilled: Defining keratin intermediate filament function in vivo." *European Journal of Cell Biology* 83(11): 735-746.

Dale, B. A., K. A. Holbrook, et al. (1985). "Expression of Epidermal Keratins and Filaggrin during Human-Fetal Skin Development." *Journal of Cell Biology* 101(4): 1257-1269.

Desmet, V. J., P. Vaneyken, et al. (1990). "Cytokeratins for Probing Cell Lineage Relationships in Developing Liver." *Hepatology* 12(5): 1249-1251.

Dinsdale, D., J. C. Lee, et al. (2004). "Intermediate filaments control the intracellular distribution of caspases during apoptosis." *American Journal of Pathology* 164(2): 395-407.

Elias, H., and Scherrick, J.C. (1969). "Microscopic anatomy of the liver." In: Morphology of the liver. H. Elias and J.C. Scherrick, eds. Academic Press, New York, pp. 1-52.

Eleazar, J. A., L. Memeo, et al. (2004). "Progenitor cell expansion: an important source of hepatocyte regeneration in chronic hepatitis." *Journal of Hepatology* 41(6): 983-991.

Fath, K. R., S. D. Obenauf, et al. (1990). "Cytoskeletal Protein and Messenger-Rna Accumulation during Brush-Border Formation in Adult Chicken Enterocytes." *Development* 109(2): 449-459.

Fickert, P., M. Trauner, et al. (2003). "Mallory body formation in primary biliary cirrhosis is associated with increased amounts and abnormal phosphorylation and ubiquitination of cytokeratins." *Journal of Hepatology* 38(4): 387-394.

Flint, N., P. W. Pemberton, et al. (1994). "Cytokeratin Expression in Epithelial-Cells Isolated from the Crypt and Villus Regions of the Rodent Small-Intestine." *Epithelial Cell Biology* 3(1): 16-23.

Fotiadu, A., V. Tzioufa, et al. (2004). "Progenitor cell activation in chronic viral hepatitis." *Liver International* 24(3): 268-274.

Gonzalez-Quintela, A., N. Mallo, et al. (2006). "Serum levels of cytokeratin-18 (tissue polypeptide-specific antigen) in liver diseases." *Liver International* 26(10): 1217-1224.

Habtezion, A., D. M. Toivola, et al. (2011). "Absence of keratin 8 confers a paradoxical microflora-dependent resistance to apoptosis in the colon." *Proceedings of the National Academy of Sciences of the United States of America* 108(4): 1445-1450.

Habtezion, A., D. M. Toivola, et al. (2005). "Keratin-8-deficient mice develop chronic spontaneous Th2 colitis amenable to antibiotic treatment." *Journal of Cell Science* 118(9): 1971-1980.

Harbaum, L., M. J. Pollheimer, et al. (2011). "Keratin 7 expression in colorectal cancer - freak of nature or significant finding?" *Histopathology* 59(2): 225-234.

Heintzelman, M. B. and M. S. Mooseker (1990). "Structural and Compositional Analysis of Early Stages in Microvillus Assembly in the Enterocyte of the Chick-Embryo." *Differentiation* 43(3): 175-182.

Herrera, M. B., S. Bruno, et al. (2006). "Isolation and characterization of a stem cell population from adult human liver." *Stem Cells* 24(12): 2840-2850.

Hesse, M., C. Grund, et al. (2007). "A mutation of keratin 18 within the coil 1A consensus motif causes widespread keratin aggregation but cell type-restricted lethality in mice." *Experimental Cell Research* 313(14): 3127-3140.

Hooper, L. V., P. G. Falk, et al. (2000). "Analyzing the molecular foundations of commensalism in the mouse intestine." *Current Opinion in Microbiology* 3(1): 79-85.

Inada, H., I. Izawa, et al. (2001). "Keratin attenuates tumor necrosis factor-induced cytotoxicity through association with TRADD." *Journal of Cell Biology* 155(3): 415-425.

Inui, A., T. Sogo, et al. (2005). "Antibodies against cytokeratin 8/18 in a patient with de novo autoimmune hepatitis after living-donor liver transplantation." *Liver Transplantation* 11(5): 504-507.

Karantza, V. (2011). "Keratins in health and cancer: more than mere epithelial cell markers." *Oncogene* 30(2): 127-138.

Khuu, D. N., M. Najimi, et al. (2007). "Epithelial cells with hepatobiliary phenotype: Is it another stem cell candidate for healthy adult human liver?" *World Journal of Gastroenterology* 13(10): 1554-1560.

Kim, S. and P. A. Coulombe (2007). "Intermediate filament scaffolds fulfill mechanical, organizational, and signaling functions in the cytoplasm." *Genes & Development* 21(13): 1581-1597.

Ku, N. O., R. Gish, et al. (2001). "Keratin 8 mutations in patients with cryptogenic liver disease." *New England Journal of Medicine* 344(21): 1580-1587.

Ku, N. O., J. Liao, et al. (1997). "Apoptosis generates stable fragments of human type I keratins." *Journal of Biological Chemistry* 272(52): 33197-33203.

Ku, N. O., S. Michie, et al. (1995). "Chronic Hepatitis, Hepatocyte Fragility, and Increased Soluble Phosphoglycokeratins in Transgenic Mice Expressing a Keratin-18 Conserved Arginine Mutant." *Journal of Cell Biology* 131(5): 1303-1314.

Ku, N. O., S. Michie, et al. (2002). "Keratin binding to 14-3-3 proteins modulates keratin filaments and hepatocyte mitotic progression." *Proceedings of the National Academy of Sciences of the United States of America* 99(7): 4373-4378.

Ku, N. O., S. A. Michie, et al. (1998). "Mutation of a major keratin phosphorylation site predisposes to hepatotoxic injury in transgenic mice." *Journal of Cell Biology* 143(7): 2023-2032.

Ku, N. O., S. A. Michie, et al. (1996). "Susceptibility to Hepatotoxicity in transgenic mice that express a dominant-negative human keratin 18 mutant." *Journal of Clinical Investigation* 98(4): 1034-1046.

Ku, N. O. and M. B. Omary (2000). "Keratins turn over by ubiquitination in a phosphorylation-modulated fashion." *Journal of Cell Biology* 149(3): 547-552.

Ku, N. O. and M. B. Omary (2006). "A disease- and phosphorylation-related nonmechanical function for keratin 8." *Journal of Cell Biology* 174(1): 115-125.

Ku, N. O., P. Strnad, et al. (2007). "Keratins let liver live: Mutations predispose to liver disease and crosslinking generates mallory-denk bodies." *Hepatology* 46(5): 1639-1649.

Ku, N. O., T. L. Wright, et al. (1997). "Mutation of human keratin 18 in association with cryptogenic cirrhosis." *Journal of Clinical Investigation* 99(1): 19-23.

Ku, N. O., X. J. Zhou, et al. (1999). "The cytoskeleton of digestive epithelia in health and disease." *American Journal of Physiology-Gastrointestinal and Liver Physiology* 277(6): G1108-G1137.

Le Naour, F., F. Brichory, et al. (2002). "A distinct repertoire of autoantibodies in hepatocellular carcinoma identified by proteomic analysis." *Molecular & Cellular Proteomics* 1(3): 197-203.

Lee, J. C., O. Schickling, et al. (2002). "DEDD regulates degradation of intermediate filaments during apoptosis." *Journal of Cell Biology* 158(6): 1051-1066.

Leers, M. P. G., W. Kolgen, et al. (1999). "Immunocytochemical detection and mapping of a cytokeratin 18 neo-epitope exposed during early apoptosis." *Journal of Pathology* 187(5): 567-572.

Li, L., S. H. Chen, et al. (2008). "Identification of hepatocellular-carcinoma-associated antigens and autoantibodies by serological proteome analysis combined with protein microarray." *Journal of Proteome Research* 7(2): 611-620.

Linder, S. (2007). "Cytokeratin markers come of age." *Tumor Biology* 28(4): 189-195.

Loranger, A., S. Duclos, et al. (1997). "Simple epithelium keratins are required for maintenance of hepatocyte integrity." *American Journal of Pathology* 151(6): 1673-1683.

Magin, T. M., R. Schroder, et al. (1998). "Lessons from keratin 18 knockout mice: Formation of novel keratin filaments, secondary loss of keratin 7 and accumulation of liver-specific keratin 8-positive aggregates." *Journal of Cell Biology* 140(6): 1441-1451.

Marceau, N., B. Schutte, et al. (2007). "Dual roles of intermediate filaments in apoptosis." *Experimental Cell Research* 313(10): 2265-2281.

Moll, R., M. Divo, et al. (2008). "The human keratins: biology and pathology." *Histochemistry and Cell Biology* 129(6): 705-733.

Moll, R., W. W. Franke, et al. (1982). "The Catalog of Human Cytokeratins - Patterns of Expression in Normal Epithelia, Tumors and Cultured-Cells." *Cell* 31(1): 11-24.

Moll, R., I. Moll, et al. (1984). "Identification of Merkel Cells in Human-Skin by Specific Cytokeratin Antibodies - Changes of Cell-Density and Distribution in Fetal and Adult Plantar Epidermis." *Differentiation* 28(2): 136-154.

Moll, R., R. Zimbelmann, et al. (1993). "The Human Gene Encoding Cytokeratin-20 and Its Expression during Fetal Development and in Gastrointestinal Carcinomas." *Differentiation* 53(2): 75-93.

Murota, M., M. Nishioka, et al. (2001). "Anti-cytokeratin antibodies in sera of the patients with autoimmune hepatitis." *Clinical and Experimental Immunology* 125(2): 291-299.

Nava, S., M. Westgren, et al. (2005). "Characterization of cells in the developing human liver." *Differentiation* 73(5): 249-260.

Omary, M. B., P. A. Coulombe, et al. (2004). "Mechanisms of disease: Intermediate filament proteins and their associated diseases." *New England Journal of Medicine* 351(20): 2087-2100.

Omary, M. B., N. O. Ku, et al. (2009). "Toward unraveling the complexity of simple epithelial keratins in human disease." *Journal of Clinical Investigation* 119(7): 1794-1805.

Oriolo, A. S., F. A. Wald, et al. (2007). "Intermediate filaments: A role in epithelial polarity." *Experimental Cell Research* 313(10): 2255-2264.

Oshima, R. G. (2002). "Apoptosis and keratin intermediate filaments." *Cell Death and Differentiation* 9(5): 486-492.

Owens, D. W. and E. B. Lane (2003). "The quest for the function of simple epithelial keratins." *Bioessays* 25(8): 748-758.

Owens, D. W. and E. B. Lane (2004). "Keratin mutations and intestinal pathology." *Journal of Pathology* 204(4): 377-385.

Owens, D. W., N. J. Wilson, et al. (2004). "Human keratin 8 mutations that disturb filament assembly observed in inflammatory bowel disease patients." *Journal of Cell Science* 117(10): 1989-1999.

Paramio, J. M. and J. L. Jorcano (2002). "Beyond structure: do intermediate filaments modulate cell signalling?" *Bioessays* 24(9): 836-844.

Pekny, M. and E. B. Lane (2007). "Intermediate filaments and stress." *Experimental Cell Research* 313(10): 2244-2254.

Quaroni, A. (1999). Role of cytokeratins in epithelial cell development. *Development of the gastrointestinal tract.* S. I. R. a. W. W. A., BC Decker Inc. 1: 57.

Quaroni, A., D. Calnek, et al. (1991). "Keratin Expression in Rat Intestinal Crypt and Villus Cells - Analysis with a Panel of Monoclonal-Antibodies." *Journal of Biological Chemistry* 266(18): 11923-11931.

Ramaekers, F., A. Huysmans, et al. (1987). "Tissue Distribution of Keratin-7 as Monitored by a Monoclonal-Antibody." *Experimental Cell Research* 170(1): 235-249.

Salas, P. J. I., M. L. Rodriguez, et al. (1997). "The apical submembrane cytoskeleton participates in the organization of the apical pole in epithelial cells." *Journal of Cell Biology* 137(2): 359-375.

Schutte, B., M. Henfling, et al. (2004). "Keratin 8/18 breakdown and reorganization during apoptosis." *Experimental Cell Research* 297(1): 11-26.

Strnad, P., R. Windoffer, et al. (2001). "In vivo detection of cytokeratin filament network breakdown in cells treated with the phosphatase inhibitor okadaic acid." *Cell and Tissue Research* 306(2): 277-293.

Tao, G. Z., I. Nakamichi, et al. (2006). "Bispecific and human disease-related anti-keratin rabbit monoclonal antibodies." *Experimental Cell Research* 312(4): 411-422.

Toivola, D. M., S. Krishnan, et al. (2004). "Keratins modulate colonocyte electrolyte transport via protein mistargeting." *Journal of Cell Biology* 164(6): 911-921.

Tot, T. (2002). "Cytokeratins 20 and 7 as biomarkers: usefulness in discriminating primary from metastatic adenocarcinoma." *European Journal of Cancer* 38(6): 758-763.

Vaneyken, P., R. Sciot, et al. (1988). "A Cytokeratin Immunohistochemical Study of Alcoholic Liver-Disease - Evidence That Hepatocytes Can Express Bile Duct-Type Cytokeratins." *Histopathology* 13(6): 605-617.

Vassy, J., T. Irinopoulou, et al. (1997). "Spatial distribution of cytoskeleton intermediate filaments during fetal rat hepatocyte differentiation." *Microscopy Research and Technique* 39(5): 436-443.

Vassy, J., M. Beil, et al. (1996). "Quantitative image analysis of cytokeratin filament distribution during fetal rat liver development." *Hepatology* 23:630-638.

Vassy, J., J. P. Rigaut, et al. (1990). "Analysis by Confocal Scanning Laser Microscopy Imaging of the Spatial-Distribution of Intermediate Filaments in Fetal and Adult-Rat Liver-Cells." *Journal of Microscopy-Oxford* 157: 91-104.

Vessey, C. J. and P. D. L. M. Hall (2001). "Hepatic stem cells: A review." *Pathology* 33(2): 130-141.

Wildi, S., J. Kleeff, et al. (1999). "Characterization of cytokeratin 20 expression in pancreatic and colorectal cancer." *Clinical Cancer Research* 5(10): 2840-2847.

Zatloukal, K., S. W. French, et al. (2007). "From Mallory to Mallory-Denk bodies: what, how and why?" *Experimental Cell Research* 313(10): 2033-2049.

Zhong, B. H., P. Strnad, et al. (2009). "Keratin Variants Are Overrepresented in Primary Biliary Cirrhosis and Associate with Disease Severity." *Hepatology* 50(2): 546-554.

Zhou, Q., M. Cadrin, et al. (2006). "Keratin 20 serine 13 phosphorylation is a stress and intestinal goblet cell marker." *Journal of Biological Chemistry* 281(24): 16453-16461.

Zhou, Q., D. M. Toivola, et al. (2003). "Keratin 20 helps maintain intermediate filament organization in intestinal epithelia." *Molecular Biology of the Cell* 14(7): 2959-2971.

Part 2

Expression of Cytokeratins in Malignant Tissues

3

Epithelial to Mesenchymal Transition in Microbial Pathogenesis

Abderrahman Chargui[1,2,**], Mimouna Sanda[1,2,**],
Patrick Brest[1,2], Paul Hofman[1,2,3] and Vouret-Craviari Valérie[1,2,*]
[1]*IRCAN, Nice,*
[2]*University of Nice-Sophia Antipolis, Nice,*
[3]*Laboratory of Clinical and Experimental Pathology and Biobank,*
Pasteur Hospital, Nice,
France

1. Introduction

Epithelia are physical barriers that constitute a functional interface between distinct body compartments and the outside. Under healthy condition, cells that composed the epithelial sheets are tightly bound to neighboring cells and to underlying basement membranes by adherens junctions, tight junctions, desmosomes and hemi-desmosomes (Farquhar, M. G. & Palade, G. E., 1963). However, epithelial cells empower high degree of plasticity and under certain circumstances such as developmental processes, fibrogenesis or tumor progression, they loss their static phenotype and acquire migratory and invasive behavior (Grunert, S., et al., 2003). Epithelial plasticity could be limited to relocalization of junctional proteins or to a more drastic epithelial to mesenchymal transition (EMT) which is characterized by disruption of intercellular contacts, loss of epithelium-specific proteins, switch to a mesenchymal gene expression pattern, and gain of invasive properties (Thiery, J. P., 2002). It is to note that EMT is different than collective cell movement which occurs when two or more cells that retain their genetic and phenotypic feature move together across a two-dimensional (layer of extracellular matrix) or through a three-dimensional interstitial tissue (Ilina, O. & Friedl, P., 2009).

2. Deciphering the EMT process

2.1 General concept

EMT has been extensively reviewed in the litterature (Nieto, M. A., 2011, Thiery, J. P., 2002, 2009) and we summarized in **Figure 1** the key point steps of this cellular process. As stated above, epithelial cells are apico-basal polarized cells with lateral adherence to their neighbors under the control of E-cadherins. The adhesion sites to extracellular matrix (ECM) are focused to the basal lamina, and cytokeratins are the main intermediate filaments. In contrast,

* Corresponding Author,
** Equal contribution

migrating mesenchymal cells display front-back polarity with only focal adhesions to their neighbors and to ECM, and have vimentin as a major intermediate filament. Therefore, loss of E-cadherin and cytokeratin and gain of vimentin are commonly used to characterize EMT.

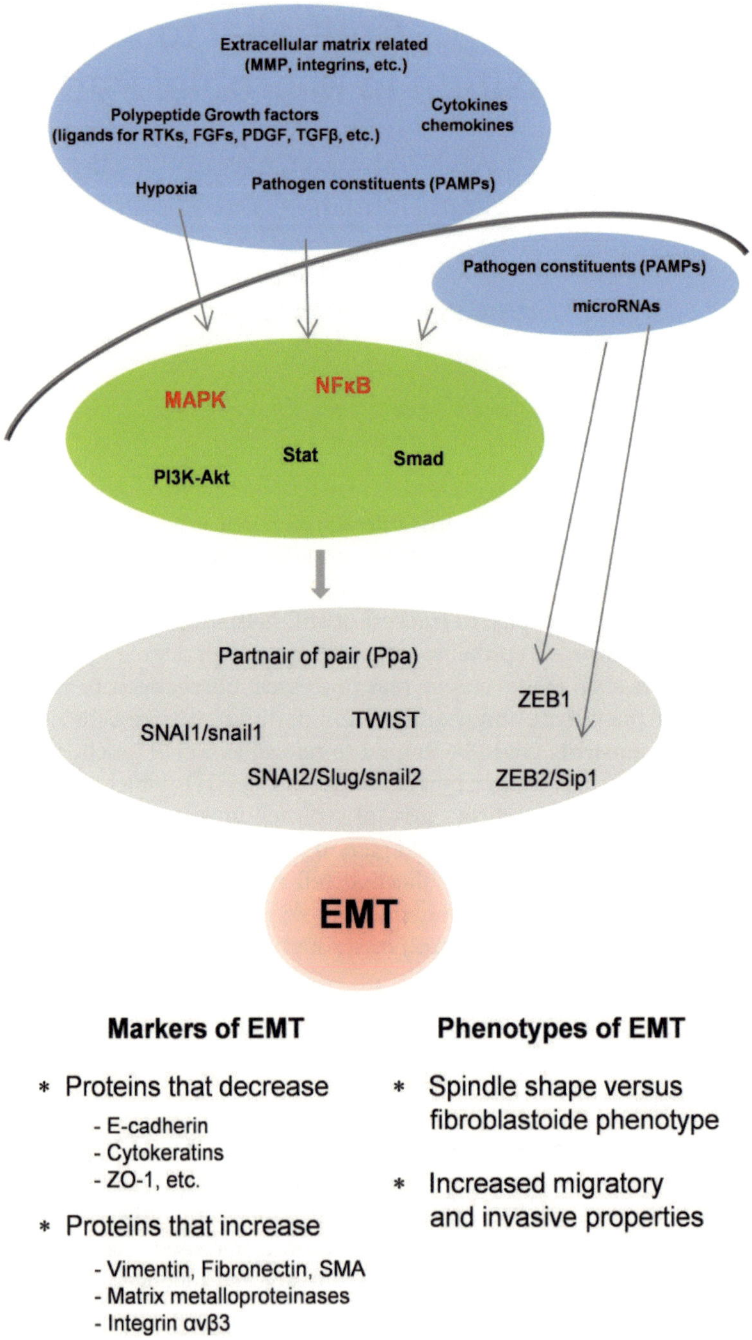

Fig. 1. A basic view of signaling pathways involved in EMT

EMT can result from various extracellular (ligands for RTKs such as FGFs, PDFG; ligands for RS/TKs such as TGFβ or ligands for specific receptors such as Wnts) and cellular stimuli (extracellular matrix compounds, hypoxia, microRNAs, ROS) that through interactions with specific receptors or other mechanisms can stimulate intracellular signaling pathways, leading to activation of transcription factors that govern the transcription of EMT-related genes. The Figure highlights NF-κB and MAPK signaling as major pathways involved in EMT triggering. The most relevant criteria to detect EMT are loss of epithelial markers (E-cadherin, Cytokeratins, ZO-1 and *etc.*) gain of mesenchymal markers (vimentin, fibronectin, MMPs, proteins of the extracellular matrix, *etc.*) associated to appearance of the fibroblastoide phenotype and increased migratory and invasive properties.

2.2 EMT and transcription factors

EMT is controlled by a small group of transcription factors defined as the core EMT regulatory factors that comprises SNAI1/Snail1 (Twigg, S. R. & Wilkie, A. O., 1999), SNAI2/Slug/Snail2 (Cohen, M. E., et al., 1998), Sip1/ZEB2 (Verschueren, K., et al., 1999) and Twist (Wang, S. M., et al., 1997). Whereas these proteins share the same function that is a transcriptional repression of E-cadherin, they have different structures. The Snail family is composed of zinc finger proteins, the ZEB family has 2 zinc finger clusters and Twist proteins has a helix loop helix motif (Peinado, H., et al., 2007). Interestingly enough, it was recently shown that in neural crest cells all these factors are coordinately regulated by an E3 ubiquitin ligase named Partner of paired (Ppa) (Lander, R., et al., 2011). Ppa is a F-box containing protein that targets its bound substrates to the ubiquitin-proteasome system for degradation. Given the importance of EMT in physiological development the existence of a common regulatory protein that can be tightly controlled in a spatio-temporal manner makes sense. However, it remains to be defined whether Ppa is also involved in pathophysiogical EMT such as tumor progression and microbial pathogenesis.

2.3 EMT and intracellular signaling pathways

Multiple signaling pathways, including receptor tyrosine kinase-mediated signals, transforming growth factor (TGF)-β/Smad, Wnt, Notch and hypoxia have been implicated as upstream initiators of the EMT process as highlighted in recent reviews (Moustakas, A. & Heldin, C. H., 2007, Peinado, H., et al., 2007, Said, N. A. & Williams, E. D., 2011). We will focus here on pathways that are activated by pathogen recognition receptors as detailed later in this review.

The MAPK module

MAPK signaling pathways are organized in modular cascades in which activation of upstream kinases by cell surface receptors leads to sequential activation of a MAPK module (MAPKKK → MAPKK → MAPK). This module comprises four different signaling pathways activated by mitogens, inflammation, stress and oxidative stress (Junttila, M. R., et al., 2008). These signaling pathways are interconnected.

The Ras>Raf>MAPK kinase cascade is activated by a large number of mitogen receptors including tyrosine kinase receptors, such as fibroblast growth factor receptor, epithelial growth factor receptor, hepatocyte growth factor, vascular endothelial growth factor and the G-protein coupled receptors, a family of seven trans-membrane domains proteins including cytokine and chemokine receptors. This signaling cascade, which is extremely well conserved from yeast to man, allows activation of a set of transcription factors which in turn control many cellular responses that are relevant for EMT (Keshet, Y. & Seger, R., 2010). Indeed, in addition to repress E-cadherin via activation of Snail/Slug, this pathway also controls upregulation of mesenchymal genes and cell motility via activation of SRE, AP1 and SP transcription factors (Grunert, S., et al., 2003) and references herein.

The p38 MAPK pathway can be activated in response to various cytokines, as well as pathogens and by environmental stress such as hypoxia. p38 MAPK was first described to down-regulate E-cadherin expression during mouse gastrulation (Zohn, I. E., et al., 2006). Further, p38 MAPK was described to participate in TNF-α (Grund, E. M., et al., 2008) and TGF-β-induced EMT (Borthwick, L. A., et al., 2011). In addition a crosstalk between the Smad and NR-κB pathways accentuates TGF-β-induced EMT in presence of TNF-α.

The c-Jun N-terminal kinase (JNK) pathway is mainly activated by cellular stress and by cytokines that act through several upstream kinases such as TAK1 and TRAF6. JNK pathway mediates TGF-β-induced EMT in keratinocytes (Santibanez, J. F., 2006). Further it was shown that activation of Smad3 by JNK is necessary to mediate TGF-β-induced EMT (Liu, Q., et al., 2008).

The Smad pathway

The best described inductor of the Smad pathway is the TGF-β that is widely described as an EMT inductor; for a review see (Zavadil, J. & Bottinger, E. P., 2005). Briefly, TGF-β binds to its receptor which then activates by phosphorylation two transcription factors, Smad-2 and Smad-3 (Massague, J., 1998). Phospho-Smad2/3 heterodimerize with Smad-4 and the Smad-complex translocate to the nucleus to regulate the transcription of genes that control cell proliferation, differentiation and cell migration (Wu, J. W., et al., 2001). Moreover, TGF-β activates Smad-independent signaling cascade leading to the activation of the classical Ras-MAPK pathway (Said, N. A. & Williams, E. D., 2011).

In addition to its well-known function in tumor progression, the TGF-β signaling plays an essential role in establishing immunological tolerance (Wan, Y. Y. & Flavell, R. A., 2007). Interestingly, reports indicate that microbe invasion lead to TGF-β modulation (Reed, S. G., 1999). First, it was shown, *in vitro* and *in vivo*, that macrophages invasion by *Trypanosoma cruzi* led to production of TGF-β (Silva, J. S., et al., 1991). This observation was then extended to bacterial infections with studies using *Mycobacterium avium* and *Mycobacterium tuberculosis* (Champsi, J., et al., 1995, Toossi, Z., et al., 1995). In the last decade it appears that many bacteria or viruses induce TGF-β production via signaling pathways that require Toll like receptors (TLR) as described below.

Macrophages represent the first line of defense; indeed most of these studies were performed on immune cells. However, TGF-β released by macrophages could activate TGF signaling on epithelial cells and then induce EMT. In agreement with this paracrine loop hypothesis, it has recently been demonstrated that increasing numbers of leukocytes (macrophages and T cells) infiltrating the kidney after acute unilateral ureteral obstruction in a mouse model correlate with increased EMT (Lange-Sperandio, B., et al., 2007).

The STAT pathway

The signal transducers and activators of transcription (STAT) family consist of seven proteins. STATs are activated by tyrosine phosphorylation of receptor tyrosine kinases, by the cytokine and chemokine receptor/Janus activated kinase (JAK) complexes or by non-receptor tyrosine kinases (Reich, N. C. & Liu, L., 2006). In general, STAT proteins have important roles in the immune response (Ihle, J. N., 2001), however STAT3 has been more particularly involved in EMT. Invalidation of the stat3 gene in mice results in early embryonic lethality (Takeda, K., et al., 1997), therefore using small interference RNA technology to efficiently block STAT3 signaling, Huang and co-authors demonstrated in pancreatic cancer cells that silencing of STAT3 resulted in suppression of EMT (Huang, C., et al., 2011).

Hypoxia

Alteration in microenvironmental oxygen tension and activation of hypoxic signaling through hypoxia-inducible factor (HIF) are emerging as important triggers and modulators of EMT (Haase, V. H., 2009, Jiang, J., et al., 2011). *In vivo*, O_2 tension varies from 2.5% to 9% in most healthy tissues. However, inflamed or diseased tissues can be deprived of O_2 (hypoxia) due to vascular damage, intensive metabolic activity of bacteria and other pathogens, and large numbers of infiltrating cells, leading to O_2 levels of less than 1%. This phenomenon results in activation of the well-coordinated mechanism leading to regulation of HIF transcriptional pathways as described in many reviews such as (Imtiyaz, H. Z., et al., 2010).

Oxygen deprivation is not the only inducer of HIF. Indeed, inflammatory cytokines, growth factors and bacterial products under normoxic conditions also induce HIFs (Blouin, C. C., et al., 2004, Cane, G., et al., 2010, Jung, Y. J., et al., 2003, Peyssonnaux, C., et al., 2008, Zhou, J., et al., 2003). Once activated HIFs, and more particularly HIF-1, controls E-cadherin repression, loss of cell-cell adhesion and cell motility via regulation of the core EMT regulatory factors in various cell types, as described in (Haase, V. H., 2009). For example, HIF-1, regulates the expression of TWIST by binding directly to the hypoxia response element in the TWIST proximal promoter (Yang, M. H., et al., 2008).

NF-κB

The NF-κB family of transcription factors which is composed of five members - p65 (REL-A), REL-B, cytoplasmic (c) REL, p50 and p52 - is widely activated under cytokines and/or microbial challenge (Li, Q. & Verma, I. M., 2002, Min, C., et al., 2008).

For example, the proinflammatory cytokines interleukin-1β and tumor necrosis factor (TNF)-α both activate and are activated by NF-κB, thus creating a positive feedback loop that results in perpetual amplification of the response.

Together with SMADs and HIF-1α, NF-κB has been shown, in an integrative genomic analysis, to regulate ZEB2, an EMT regulator, (Katoh, M., 2009). In addition, NF-κB is involved in the up regulation of *twist-1* and *twist-2* expression in response to TNF-α; this regulation is lost in fibroblasts lacking the p65 subunit of NF-κB (Sosic, D., et al., 2003). Moreover, the authors proposed a model in which TWIST orchestrates a negative feedback loop by repressing cytokine expression under cytokine challenge and therefore maintaining a controlled inflammatory response.

Interestingly enough, the classical NF-κB pathway is also responsible for the EMT process attributable to *Von Hippel-Lindau* (VHL) loss and subsequent HIF-1 activation since molecular and pharmacological approaches to inhibit NF-κB promote a partial reversion to an epithelial phenotype (Pantuck, A. J., et al., 2010).

Finally, NF-κB also controls mesenchymal marker expression. The NF-kB binding site has been described on the vimentin gene (Lilienbaum, A., et al., 1990) and overexpression of a constitutively active form of p65 in breast cancer cells increases expression of vimentin (Chua, H. L., et al., 2007). Moreover, NF-κB directly activates the transcription of the matrix metalloprotease (MMP)-9 gene, a type IV collagenase which increases cellular invasiveness and motility (Himelstein, B. P., et al., 1997) and indirectly controls MMP-2 (Yoshizaki, T., et al., 2002).

MicroRNAs

MicroRNAs (miRs) are non-coding RNA of 18-24 bp that post transcriptionally regulate gene expression. The key region of miRs that governs their target specificity, named the seed sequence, encompasses bases 2-7 from their 5′ end (Lewis, B. P., et al., 2005). More than 1200 miRNAs have been identified in humans, and each individual miR could regulate ten to hundreds of genes according to the presence of seed sequence matches in their 3′UTRs. The ability of a specific miR to modify gene expression is governed by its seed sequence but also its expression, which could be spatiotemporally regulated.

A microRNA microarray profiling performed on MDCK undergoing EMT allowed to characterize the implication of the miR-200 family (miR-200a, miR-200b, miR-200c, miR-141 and miR-429) and miR-205. Decrease in expression of each of these miRs correlates with decreased expression of E-cadherin and increases in mesenchymal markers mRNA such as vimentin and fibronectin. In addition, overexpression of these miRs in MDCK cells prevents EMT demonstrating that down-regulation of these miRs is an essential component of the EMT process. Finally, it was shown that the miR-200 family represses endogenous expression of ZEB1 and ZEB2 (Bracken, C. P., et al., 2008, Gregory, P. A., et al., 2008, Korpal, M., et al., 2008, Park, S. M., et al., 2008).

As mentioned previously in this report, TGFβ is a powerful inductor of EMT. A combination of miRs and mRNA profiling was used to identify miRs that destabilize mRNAs in TGFβ-directed EMT. Such strategy allowed the characterization of eight miRs specific of a particular signature of EMT-like response (Zavadil, J., et al., 2007).

3. Pattern recognition receptor-induced signaling pathways

3.1 A general overview on PRR

Charles Janeway was the first to understand that recognition of pathogen-associated molecular patterns (PAMPs) by host pathogen-recognition receptors (PRRs) is the basis of immune immunity and represents the first defense against pathogens (Janeway, C. A., Jr., 1989). His discovery was further confirmed by the identification of Toll-like receptor (TLR)4 as the protein involved in the recognition of lipopolysaccharide (LPS), therefore making the link between a microbial motif, LPS, and a host receptor, TLR4 (Poltorak, A., et al., 1998). A new axe of researches was then opened and after more than a decade the TLRs family encounters 10 members in human and each TLR has a distinct function in terms of PAMP recognition (Kawai, T. & Akira, S., 2010).

TLRs are divided into two subgroups based on their cellular localization and respective PAMP ligands. The first group, expressed on cell surfaces which recognize mainly microbial membrane components such as lipids, lipoproteins and proteins, is composed of TLR1, TLR2, TLR4, TLR5, TLR6 and TLR11; the second group, expressed exclusively in intracellular vesicles where the receptors recognize microbial nucleic acids, is composed of TLR3, TLR7, TLR8 and TLR9.

In mammals, in addition to TLRs, an intra-cytoplasmic sensing system for microbial effector exists. This second family of receptors is named Nod (nucleotide-binding oligomerization domain)-like receptors (NLRs); NLRs sense the presence of intracellular muropeptides (Fritz, J. H., et al., 2006). As highlighted in **Figure 2** both TLRs and NLRs activate intracellular signaling pathways that share common adaptors with receptors of growth factors, cytokines or chemokines.

Note that in addition to TLRs and NLRs other microbial sensors exist as reviewed in (Bouchon, A., et al., 2000, Crocker, P. R., 2005, Klesney-Tait, J., et al., 2006, Robinson, M. J., et al., 2006).

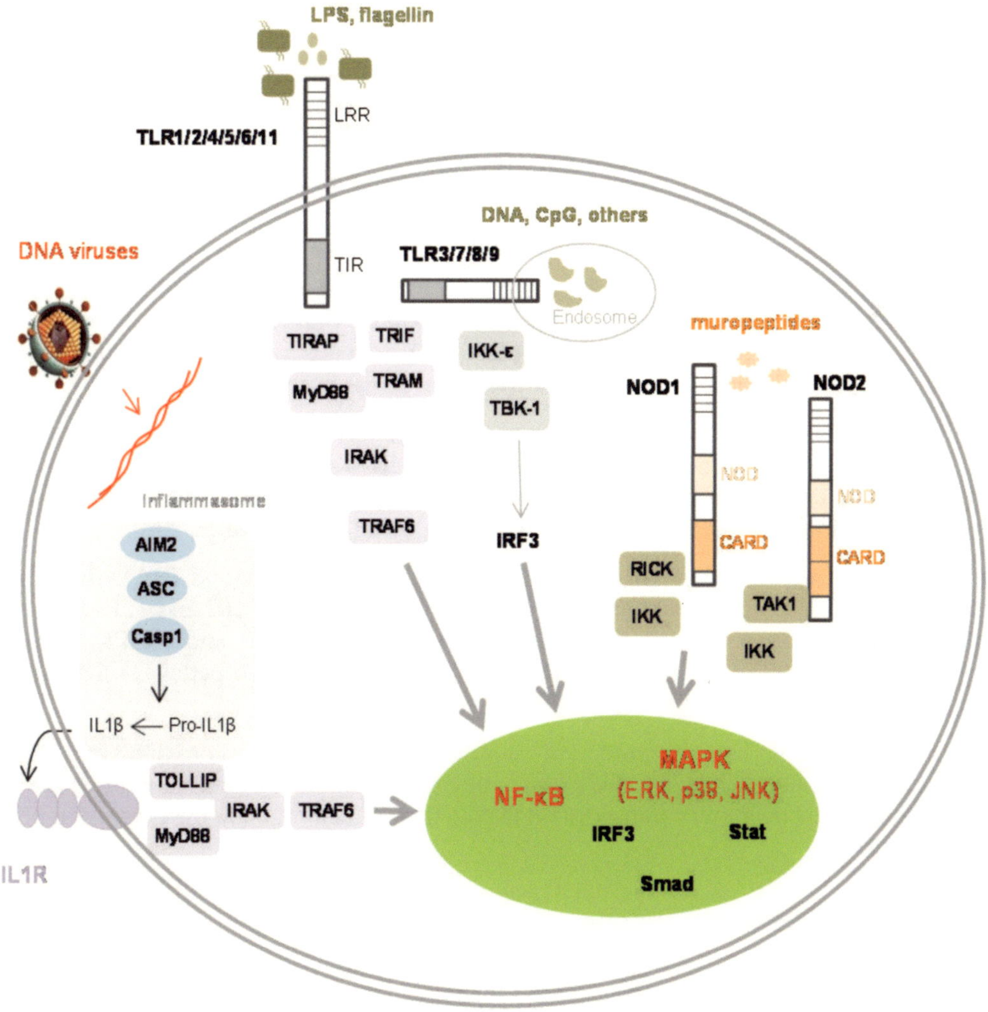

Fig. 2. A schematic view of PPR-induced pathways involved in stimulation of NF-κB and MAPK signaling

TLRs (TLR1, TLR2, TLR4, TLR5, TLR6, TLR7 and TLR9) do activate NF-κB and MAPK module - comprising ERK, p38 and JNK - by binding of MyD88 to the receptor TIR domain and subsequently triggering IRAK, TRAF6 and TAK1 which ultimately activate the IkB kinase (IKK) complex - which consists of IKK-α, IKK-β and IKK-γ (also known as IKK1,

IKK2 and nuclear factor-κB (NF-κB) essential modulator, NEMO, respectively - and MAPKs. Alternatively, TIRAP (TIR domain-containing adaptor protein), a second TIR-domain-containing adaptor protein, is involved in the MyD88-dependent signalling pathway through TLR2 and TLR4. A third TIR-domain-containing adaptor, TRIF (TIR domain-containing adaptor protein inducing IFN-β), is essential for the MyD88-independent pathway. Further, the non-typical IKKs IKK-ε and TBK1 (TRAF-family-member-associated NF-κB activator (TANK)-binding kinase 1) mediate activation of IRF3 downstream of TRIF. A fourth TIR-domain containing adaptor, TRAM (TRIF-related adaptor molecule), is specific to the TLR4-mediated, MyD88-independent/TRIF-dependent pathway. By contrast, activation of NLRs leads to the recruitment of the receptor-interacting protein 2 (RIP2) kinase, which is essential for the activation of the IKK complex. In addition, activation of NOD1 leads to JNK stimulation. Finally, double strand DNA has been linked to inflammasome activation. This protein complex which is composed of NLRs of the NALP-family and adaptor-proteins apoptosis-associated speck-like protein (ASC), mediates the generation of IL-1β through cleavage of its precursor by caspase-1.

3.2 PRR and mediators of EMT

TLRs are type I trans-membrane proteins with extracellular domains containing leucine-rich repeats and mediating the recognition of PAMPs, trans-membrane domains and intracellular Toll–interleukin 1 (IL-1) receptor (TIR) domains which recruit TIR domain-containing adaptor molecules to induce downstream signal transduction.

MyD88 was identified as the first member of the TIR family adaptors. Once bound to TLRs, MyD88 recruits the IL-1 receptor–associated kinases IRAK4, IRAK1, IRAK2 and IRAK-M. Mostly, direct or indirect activation of IRAK allows the activation of NF-κB and MAPK which in turn induces various transcription factors (Kawai, T. & Akira, S., 2010).

The TIR family also comprise TIRAP (Mal), TRAM and TRIF. TIRAP and TRAM function as additional sorting adaptors allowing the recruitment of MyD88 to TLR2 and TLR4. The final consequence of this signaling puzzle is the activation of NF-κB and MAPK signaling pathways. TRIF is used by TLR3 and TLR4 and induces alternative pathways that lead to activation of the transcription factors IRF3 and NF-κB

Interestingly enough, host recognition of pathogens lead to activation of NF-κB and MAPK pathways. As mentioned earlier, these two pathways are particularly relevant for EMT since they control the activation of transcription factors that in turn regulate the expression of the EMT core genes.

4. EMT and bacterial pathogens

The microbes normally present in humans are collectively estimated to number tenfold that of human cells. Mainly located in the gut, the microbiota is crucial for human life by influencing human physiology and nutriment uptake (Ley, R. E., et al., 2006). In addition, the microbiota contributes to the shaping of healthy intestinal immune responses (Inagaki, H., et al., 1996). It has been proposed that an alteration in the development and/or composition of the microbiota may disturb the relationship between microbes and the immune system. In turn, immune defects may favor pathogenesis of various human inflammatory disorders (Round, J. L. & Mazmanian, S. K., 2009) and inflammatory disorders promote EMT.

We can therefore speculate that most of microbes that persist in the body have the potential to indirectly favor an EMT behavior. In this review we will only focus on the few examples that describe a direct involvement of microbial pathogens in EMT induction.

4.1 Lipopolysaccharide

Lipopolysaccharide (LPS) is the major component of the outer membrane of Gram-negative bacteria. LPS is an endotoxin which induces a strong response from normal animal immune systems; therefore it is widely used to study gram-negative bacteria-induced cellular responses. Intriguingly, we found in the literature only one report that studies LPS-induced EMT. Using a model of intrahepatic biliary epithelial cells, Zhao and co-authors have shown that in response to LPS stimulation a decrease in E-cadherin expression was observed whereas expression of the mesenchymal markers (S100A and α–SMA) increased by more than 12-fold (Zhao, L., et al., 2010). In addition to EMT markers, they noticed that the messenger coding for TGFβ-1 was significantly increased. As indicated previously, TGFβ-1 is a well-known inductor of EMT that transmits its effect via Smad2/3. Indeed, silencing of Smad 2/3 in biliary epithelial cells resulted in a significant decrease of mesenchymal markers and an increase in E-cadherin expression. Therefore, the authors concluded that LPS induced the EMT probably through the TGF-β1/Smad2/3 pathway.

4.2 *Helicobacter pylori*

Helicobacter pylori is a gram-negative bacteria which colonizes the human stomach of about 50% of the world's population. Although a large proportion of infected subjects can develop gastritis, 80% of these individuals remain asymptomatic. Severe *H. pylori*-mediated diseases are duodenal and gastric ulcer disease, gastric cancer and mucosa-associated lymphoid tissues (MALT) lymphomas affecting about 15%, 1% and 0.1% of infected people, respectively (Amieva, M. R. & El-Omar, E. M., 2008). Since 1994, *H. pylori* is classified as a class I carcinogen by the World Health Organization. More than 350 genetically different strains have been identified. To avoid mechanical clearance, *H. pylori* first adhere to the gastric epithelium due to adhesins. Among their numerous virulence factors, the two major virulence factors of *H. pylori*, the cytotoxin VacA and the cag pathogenicity island and its effector CagA, can co-opt epithelial cell function. Whereas VacA can disrupt the barrier function of tight junction, it does not perturb junction integrity (Papini, E., et al., 1998), CagA has major effects on the apical junctional complex allowing the deregulation of epithelial cell-cell adhesion and a loss in epithelial polarity (Amieva, M. R., et al., 2003, Murata-Kamiya, N., et al., 2007).

Using the pathogenic H. Pylori strain 60190, Yin and co-authors observed expression of Snail and Slug in gastric epithelial cells (Yin, Y., et al., 2010). Further, they demonstrated that induction of EMT genes depends on *H. pylori*-induced signaling cascade pathways that involve gastrin, MMP7 and shedding of soluble heparin-binding epidermal growth factor. Interestingly, the increase of gastrin observed in response to *H. pylori* infection occurred via a Ras>Raf>Mek>Erk>NF-κb signaling pathway (Brandt, S., et al., 2005). Then, it appears that NF-κB is a central common effector that plays a key role in the EMT process.

As mentioned earlier, HIFs are also involved in EMT regulation. It is noteworthy that ROS stabilize HIF-1α (Park, J. H., et al., 2003) and *H. pylori* induce ROS (Bagchi, D., et al., 1996).

Therefore, one could speculate that *H. pylori*-induced stabilization of HIF-1 acts in combination with NF-κB to maximally induce the EMT program.

4.3 Enterovirulent *Escherichia coli* strains

Escherichia coli which colonize the gastrointestinal tract of human infants within a few hours after birth normally coexist in harmony with its human hosts. However, there are several highly adapted *E. coli* clones that have acquired specific virulence factors, which confer an increased ability to adapt to new niches and allow them to cause a broad spectrum of diseases. Among the intestinal pathogens there are six well described classes: enteropathogenic-, enterohaemorrhagic-, enterotoxigenic-, enteroaggregative-, enteroinvasive- and diffusely adherent-*E. coli*. Enteropathogenic *E. coli* cause entero/diarrhoeal disease as a consequence of lack of intestinal barrier permeability (Kaper, J. B., et al., 2004). In most of the cases this epithelial plasticity is limited to relocalization of junctional proteins; however, depending on the bacterial strain used to infect epithelial cells, it could lead to a more drastic EMT.

Among the families of entero-pathogenic *E. coli*, diffusely adherent *E. coli* (DAEC) is a heterogeneous group with variable virulence factors promoting adherence to epithelial cells (Servin, A. L., 2005) The pathogenicity of such bacteria is still controversial; however, the presence of DAEC expressing Afa/Dr adhesins has been reported in epidemiological studies of various types of enterocolitis (Meraz, I. M., et al., 2007, Vargas, M., et al., 1998). Afa/Dr DAEC strains are a family of DAEC expressing the afimbrial Afa-I and Afa-III adhesins, Dr haemagglutinin and fimbrial F1845 adhesin. Afa/Dr adhesins interact with receptors such as the membrane-associated decay accelerating factor (DAF/ CD55), the carcino-embryonic-antigen (CEA/CD66e) and CEACAM-1, -3, -6 (Berger, C. N., et al., 2004), leading to cell signaling. Using the clinical isolate DAEC C1845, we have shown that infection of intestinal epithelial cells promotes EMT-like behavior. We have deciphered the molecular mechanisms leading to EMT and observed that F1845 adhesin binding to the DAF receptor promotes Ras>Raf>MAPK and PI3K pathways (Betis, F., et al., 2003a, 2003b, Cane, G., et al., 2007). Activation of these signaling pathways is required to induce an increase in HIF-1α protein expression but also Twist1 mRNA expression. We noticed that HIF-1α silencing significantly blocked the expression of Twist1 gene, revealing a role for HIF-1 in the transcriptional regulation of this gene. Furthermore, we observed that C1845-induced HIF-1α protein expression leads to a loss of E-cadherin and cytokeratin 18 and an increase in fibronectin expression, which are reversed in HIF-1α silenced cells (Cane, G., et al., 2010), therefore highlighting the critical role of HIF in DAEC-induced EMT.

5. EMT and viral pathogens

As for microbial pathogens, viral infection leads to activation of intracellular signaling pathways (Rathinam, V. A. & Fitzgerald, K. A., 2011); thus we can intuitively speculate that viruses can induce EMT. The major pathogenic viruses include cytomegalovirus (CMV), herpes simplex virus (HSV), Epstein–Barr virus, Kaposi's sarcoma-associated herpes virus, polyoma virus, hepatitis B and C virus and human papilloma virus. Previous works indeed confirmed that at least two families of viruses (Epstein-barr and hepatitis B and C) induce EMT in epithelial cells.

5.1 Epstein-barr virus

Epstein–Barr virus (EBV) is a member of the herpes virus family which infects more than 90% of world population. EBV utilizes normal B cell biology to infect, persist, and replicate in B cells. Beyond immune cells, EBV also infects epithelial cells and it has been associated with neoplastic diseases such as nasopharyngeal carcinoma (Chen, M.-R., 2011); the link between EBV and EMT has been studied in this particular context.

Latent EBV encodes for eight proteins, two of them, the latent membrane protein 1 and 2A (LMPs), which highjack cell host signaling (Caldwell, R. G., et al., 1998, Gires, O., et al., 1997), are particularly involved in EMT. Horikawa and coauthors were the first to describe that transformation of MDCK epithelial cells with LMP1 induces EMT, characterized by loss of epithelial markers, gain of mesenchymal markers and its associated increase in cell motility and invasiveness (Horikawa, T., et al., 2007). To go further, the authors have shown that Twist1-silencing in MDCK cells resulted in changes from scattered and fibroblast-like shapes to tightly packed cobblestone morphology, characteristics of mesenchymal-to-epithelial transition, the reverse of EMT. Finally, the authors demonstrated that LMP1 induces Twist through NF-κB in nasopharyngeal epithelial cells. More recently the same group demonstrated that Snail1 acts in combination to twist1 to induce EMT in nasopharyngeal carcinoma cells (Horikawa, T., et al., 2011).

Using nasopharyngeal carcinoma tumor samples the group of Zeng has shown that 57.6% of tumors overexpressed LMP2A at the tumor invasive front (Kong, Q. L., et al., 2010). Interestingly enough, LMP2A increases the size of the stem-like cell population and the number of tumor initial cells; this effect being reversed by inhibitors of AKT.

In addition to a classical effect on intracellular signaling, EBV also down regulates expression of miR-200a and miR-200b, the down regulation of which induces EMT (Shinozaki, A., et al., 2010). First, the authors demonstrated an association between miR-200a and miR-200b down regulation and E-cadherin expression on resected gastric carcinoma tissue. Further, using *in vitro* established EBV-infected cell lines they confirmed that down regulation of these miRs correlates with up regulation the ZEB family of transcription factors and their associated loss of cell-to-cell adhesion. Finally they uncovered the ability of LMP2A, EBNA1 and BARF0 to down regulate the pri-miR-200 transcript.

EBV is found in alveolar epithelial cells where it is suspected to promote idiopathic pulmonary fibrosis. Indeed, active EVB infection regulates EMT in alveolar epithelial cells (Malizia, A. P., et al., 2009). In this report the authors highlighted the role of Wnt signaling, since Wnt5B-silenced cells are resistant to EBV-induced EMT. Further, using an *ex vivo* cell system model the authors demonstrated that activation of non-canonical Wnt signaling pathway by EBV is dependent of CUX1 signaling. Therefore a link between EBV and fibrosis was demonstrated with EMT being the core of the process. This former observation was recently confirmed and extended. Indeed, the group of Lasky demonstrated that LMP1 induces pro-EMT signaling that occurs primarily through the nuclear factor-κB pathway and secondarily through the extracellular signal-regulated kinase (ERK) pathway (Sides, M. D., et al., 2011).

5.2 Hepatitis B and C viruses

At least seven different viruses cause hepatitis, hepatitis viruses A, B and C are the most known. Whereas hepatitis virus A (HAV) induces acute infection disease of the liver, HBV and HCV induce more chronic diseases that can lead to cirrhosis and hepatocellular carcinoma. Both HBV and HCV have been shown to induce EMT.

Viral particles of mammalian HBV encode for a small regulatory protein, known as the X protein that modulates intracellular signaling pathways by directly or indirectly interacting with host factors. Therefore it was hypothesized that HBV X protein may induce EMT in hepatocytes. To test this hypothesis Yang and coauthors transfected hepatocytes with HBx gene and observed that cells underwent morphological changes from an epithelial morphology to spindle-like shape associated with an increase in invasive potential (Yang, S. Z., et al., 2009). When the authors treated the cells with PP2, a well-known inhibitor of the Src kinase family, they noticed that cells recovered their original epithelial morphology. Therefore, they claimed that activated c-Src played a critical role in the HBx-induced EMT of hepatocytes.

HCV core protein which interacts with various cellular proteins induces host cells responses (Delhem, N., et al., 2001, Lai, M. M. & Ware, C. F., 2000, Zhu, N., et al., 1998). Of particular interest, HCV core protein interacts with Smad3 and consequently inhibits TGF-β induced Smad3 transcriptional activity (Pavio, N., et al., 2005). Since the TGF-β/Smad3 pathway induces EMT, it was suspected that HCV core protein directly impacts on the EMT process. Using stably transfected cell lines and primary mouse hepatocytes, as well as primary human hepatocytes infected *in vitro* with lentiviruses encoding HCV core protein, Battaglia and coauthors demonstrated that core protein expression was sufficient to provoke EMT in primary hepatocytes. This effect was reverted by addition of a specific inhibitor of TGF-β I receptor thus demonstrating a TGF-β dependent effect of core on EMT development (Battaglia, S., et al., 2009).

HCV core protein has also been involved in the pathogenesis of cholangiocarcinoma. In agreement with this idea, HCV core protein expression in cholangiocarcinoma cells induces EMT through a mechanism dependent on LOXL2 pathway (Li, T., et al., 2010).

6. Perspective: EMT and microbial pathogenesis

The field of research encompassing EMT has been one of the most exciting areas in embryogenesis, organ development, wound repair and tissue remodeling over the past 10 years. This overview is by no means intended to provide a global view on EMT. Instead, as shown in **Figure 3**, we have attempted to depict the main lines which govern EMT in order to highlight similarities that exist between growth factor-and pathogens-induced signaling pathways allowing us to give a coherent picture of the place of microbial infection in EMT and subsequent human pathologies. However, it is important to note that in healthy individuals, infection is effectively controlled, and the inflammatory response is promptly resolved. Indeed, microbes-induced chronic inflammation is intimately linked to defective innate immunity correlating with microenvironment, genetic and epigenetic susceptibilities but also treatment access. For example, *H. pylori* colonize the human stomach of about 50% of the world's population, however less than 2% of this population will develop a stomack cancer, implying the existence of individual predispositon.

Interestingly, it appears that only pathogens associated to chronic pathologies (fibrinogenesis, cancer) (Hofman, P. M., 2010) have been described to induce EMT. Given that all pathogen recognition receptors induce NF-κB and MAPK module, one can speculate that each pathogen may have the potential to induce EMT as for as its attack remains unresolved by innate immunity. Keeping that in mind, we can assume that a large part of EMT knowledge can be moved to translational research in molecular medicine with potential future new therapeutics in treating diseases linked to infections.

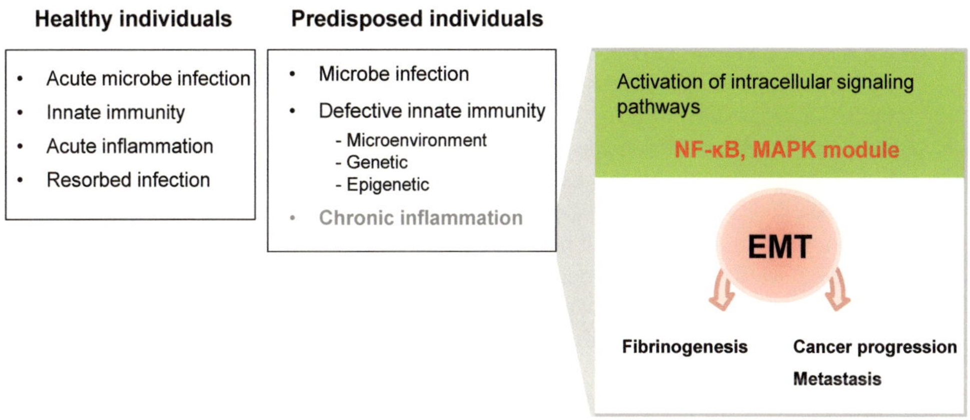

Fig. 3. Microbe-induced chronic inflammation in predisposed individuals leads to EMT

Here we suggest a model in which microbe infection plays a critical role as an EMT promoter. In healthy individuals, microbe infection is contained by the innate immunity. By contrast in predisposed individuals the innate immunity is exceeded by microbe infection leading to chronic inflammation. Chronic inflammation, associated to chronic infection lead to sustained NF-κB and MAPK module activation: the basement of EMT. Finally, EMT plays a critical role in onset of various human pathologies such as fibrinogenesis, cancer progression and metastasis.

7. Acknowledgment

We thank L. Bianchini for her critical feedback and thoughtful suggestions. We apologize to those investigators whose experimental work has not been cited or cited indirectly owing to space limitations. Experimental work was supported by the «Institut National de la Santé et de la Recherche Médicale», the « Centre National de la Recherche Scientifique », the « Ministère de l'Education, de la Recherche et de la Technologie », and by grants from « Association pour la Recherche sur le Cancer » (ARC, subvention 1142), « Association François Aupetit » and « Fondation Infectiopole Sud ».

8. References

M. G. Farquhar & G. E. Palade (1963). Junctional complexes in various epithelia, *J Cell Biol,* Vol.17, pp.375-412, ISSN 0021-9525

S. Grunert, M. Jechlinger & H. Beug (2003). Diverse cellular and molecular mechanisms contribute to epithelial plasticity and metastasis, *Nat Rev Mol Cell Biol,* Vol.4, No.8, pp.657-65, ISSN 1471-0072

J. P. Thiery (2002). Epithelial-mesenchymal transitions in tumour progression, *Nat Rev Cancer,* Vol.2, No.6, pp.442-54, ISSN 1474-175X

O. Ilina & P. Friedl (2009). Mechanisms of collective cell migration at a glance, *J Cell Sci,* Vol.122, No.Pt 18, pp.3203-8, ISSN 1477-9137

M. A. Nieto (2011). the ins and outs of the epithelial to mesenchymal transition in health and disease, *Annual review Cell Dev Biol,* Vol.in press

J. P. Thiery, H. Acloque, R. Y. Huang & M. A. Nieto (2009). Epithelial-mesenchymal transitions in development and disease, *Cell,* Vol.139, No.5, pp.871-90, ISSN 1097-4172

S. R. Twigg & A. O. Wilkie (1999). Characterisation of the human snail (SNAI1) gene and exclusion as a major disease gene in craniosynostosis, *Hum Genet,* Vol.105, No.4, pp.320-6, ISSN 0340-6717

M. E. Cohen, M. Yin, W. A. Paznekas, M. Schertzer, S. Wood & E. W. Jabs (1998). Human SLUG gene organization, expression, and chromosome map location on 8q, *Genomics,* Vol.51, No.3, pp.468-71, ISSN 0888-7543

K. Verschueren, J. E. Remacle, C. Collart, H. Kraft, B. S. Baker, P. Tylzanowski, L. Nelles, G. Wuytens, M. T. Su, R. Bodmer, J. C. Smith & D. Huylebroeck (1999). SIP1, a novel zinc finger/homeodomain repressor, interacts with Smad proteins and binds to 5'-CACCT sequences in candidate target genes, *J Biol Chem,* Vol.274, No.29, pp.20489-98, ISSN 0021-9258

S. M. Wang, V. W. Coljee, R. J. Pignolo, M. O. Rotenberg, V. J. Cristofalo & F. Sierra (1997). Cloning of the human twist gene: its expression is retained in adult mesodermally-derived tissues, *Gene,* Vol.187, No.1, pp.83-92, ISSN 0378-1119

H. Peinado, D. Olmeda & A. Cano (2007). Snail, Zeb and bHLH factors in tumour progression: an alliance against the epithelial phenotype?, *Nat Rev Cancer,* Vol.7, No.6, pp.415-28, ISSN 1474-175X

R. Lander, K. Nordin & C. Labonne (2011). The F-box protein Ppa is a common regulator of core EMT factors Twist, Snail, Slug, and Sip1, *J Cell Biol,* Vol.194, No.1, pp.17-25, ISSN 1540-8140

A. Moustakas & C. H. Heldin (2007). Signaling networks guiding epithelial-mesenchymal transitions during embryogenesis and cancer progression, *Cancer Sci,* Vol.98, No.10, pp.1512-20, ISSN 1347-9032

N. A. Said & E. D. Williams (2011). Growth factors in induction of epithelial-mesenchymal transition and metastasis, *Cells Tissues Organs,* Vol.193, No.1-2, pp.85-97, ISSN 1422-6421

M. R. Junttila, S. P. Li & J. Westermarck (2008). Phosphatase-mediated crosstalk between MAPK signaling pathways in the regulation of cell survival, *FASEB J,* Vol.22, No.4, pp.954-65, ISSN 1530-6860

Y. Keshet & R. Seger (2010). The MAP kinase signaling cascades: a system of hundreds of components regulates a diverse array of physiological functions, *Methods Mol Biol,* Vol.661, pp.3-38, ISSN 1940-6029

I. E. Zohn, Y. Li, E. Y. Skolnik, K. V. Anderson, J. Han & L. Niswander (2006). p38 and a p38-interacting protein are critical for downregulation of E-cadherin during mouse gastrulation, *Cell,* Vol.125, No.5, pp.957-69, ISSN 0092-8674

E. M. Grund, D. Kagan, C. A. Tran, A. Zeitvogel, A. Starzinski-Powitz, S. Nataraja & S. S. Palmer (2008). Tumor necrosis factor-alpha regulates inflammatory and mesenchymal responses via mitogen-activated protein kinase kinase, p38, and nuclear factor kappaB in human endometriotic epithelial cells, *Mol Pharmacol,* Vol.73, No.5, pp.1394-404, ISSN 1521-0111

L. A. Borthwick, A. Gardner, A. De Soyza, D. A. Mann & A. J. Fisher (2011). Transforming Growth Factor-beta1 (TGF-beta1) Driven Epithelial to Mesenchymal Transition (EMT) is Accentuated by Tumour Necrosis Factor alpha (TNFalpha) via Crosstalk Between the SMAD and NF-kappaB Pathways, *Cancer Microenviron,* ISSN 1875-2284 J. F. Santibanez (2006). JNK mediates TGF-beta1-induced epithelial mesenchymal transdifferentiation of mouse transformed keratinocytes, *FEBS Lett,* Vol.580, No.22, pp.5385-91, ISSN 0014-5793

Q. Liu, H. Mao, J. Nie, W. Chen, Q. Yang, X. Dong & X. Yu (2008). Transforming growth factor {beta}1 induces epithelial-mesenchymal transition by activating the JNK-Smad3 pathway in rat peritoneal mesothelial cells, *Perit Dial Int,* Vol.28 Suppl 3, pp.S88-95, ISSN 0896-8608

J. Zavadil & E. P. Bottinger (2005). TGF-beta and epithelial-to-mesenchymal transitions, *Oncogene,* Vol.24, No.37, pp.5764-74, ISSN 0950-9232

J. Massague (1998). TGF-beta signal transduction, *Annu Rev Biochem,* Vol.67, pp.753-91, ISSN 0066-4154

J. W. Wu, M. Hu, J. Chai, J. Seoane, M. Huse, C. Li, D. J. Rigotti, S. Kyin, T. W. Muir, R. Fairman, J. Massague & Y. Shi (2001). Crystal structure of a phosphorylated Smad2. Recognition of phosphoserine by the MH2 domain and insights on Smad function in TGF-beta signaling, *Mol Cell,* Vol.8, No.6, pp.1277-89, ISSN 1097-2765

Y. Y. Wan & R. A. Flavell (2007). 'Yin-Yang' functions of transforming growth factor-beta and T regulatory cells in immune regulation, *Immunol Rev,* Vol.220, pp.199-213, ISSN 0105-2896 S. G. Reed (1999). TGF-beta in infections and infectious diseases, *Microbes Infect,* Vol.1, No.15, pp.1313-25, ISSN 1286-4579

J. S. Silva, D. R. Twardzik & S. G. Reed (1991). Regulation of Trypanosoma cruzi infections in vitro and in vivo by transforming growth factor beta (TGF-beta), *J Exp Med,* Vol.174, No.3, pp.539-45, ISSN 0022-1007

J. Champsi, L. S. Young & L. E. Bermudez (1995). Production of TNF-alpha, IL-6 and TGF-beta, and expression of receptors for TNF-alpha and IL-6, during murine Mycobacterium avium infection, *Immunology,* Vol.84, No.4, pp.549-54, ISSN 0019-2805

Z. Toossi, T. G. Young, L. E. Averill, B. D. Hamilton, H. Shiratsuchi & J. J. Ellner (1995). Induction of transforming growth factor beta 1 by purified protein derivative of Mycobacterium tuberculosis, *Infect Immun,* Vol.63, No.1, pp.224-8, ISSN 0019-9567

B. Lange-Sperandio, A. Trautmann, O. Eickelberg, A. Jayachandran, S. Oberle, F. Schmidutz, B. Rodenbeck, M. Homme, R. Horuk & F. Schaefer (2007). Leukocytes induce epithelial to mesenchymal transition after unilateral ureteral obstruction in neonatal mice, *Am J Pathol,* Vol.171, No.3, pp.861-71, ISSN 0002-9440

N. C. Reich & L. Liu (2006). Tracking STAT nuclear traffic, *Nat Rev Immunol,* Vol.6, No.8, pp.602-12, ISSN 1474-1733 (Print)

1474-1733 (Linking)

J. N. Ihle (2001). The Stat family in cytokine signaling, *Curr Opin Cell Biol,* Vol.13, No.2, pp.211-7, ISSN 0955-0674

K. Takeda, K. Noguchi, W. Shi, T. Tanaka, M. Matsumoto, N. Yoshida, T. Kishimoto & S. Akira (1997). Targeted disruption of the mouse Stat3 gene leads to early embryonic lethality, *Proc Natl Acad Sci U S A,* Vol.94, No.8, pp.3801-4, ISSN 0027-8424

C. Huang, G. Yang, T. Jiang, G. Zhu, H. Li & Z. Qiu (2011). The effects and mechanisms of blockage of STAT3 signaling pathway on IL-6 inducing EMT in human pancreatic cancer cells in vitro, *Neoplasma,* Vol.58, No.5, pp.396-405, ISSN 0028-2685

V. H. Haase (2009). Oxygen regulates epithelial-to-mesenchymal transition: insights into molecular mechanisms and relevance to disease, *Kidney Int,* Vol.76, No.5, pp.492-9, ISSN 1523-1755

J. Jiang, Y. L. Tang & X. H. Liang (2011). EMT: a new vision of hypoxia promoting cancer progression, *Cancer Biol Ther,* Vol.11, No.8, pp.714-23, ISSN 1555-8576

H. Z. Imtiyaz, E. P. Williams, M. M. Hickey, S. A. Patel, A. C. Durham, L. J. Yuan, R. Hammond, P. A. Gimotty, B. Keith & M. C. Simon (2010). Hypoxia-inducible factor 2alpha regulates macrophage function in mouse models of acute and tumor inflammation, *J Clin Invest,* Vol.120, No.8, pp.2699-714, ISSN 1558-8238

C. C. Blouin, E. L. Page, G. M. Soucy & D. E. Richard (2004). Hypoxic gene activation by lipopolysaccharide in macrophages: implication of hypoxia-inducible factor 1alpha, *Blood,* Vol.103, No.3, pp.1124-30, ISSN 0006-4971

G. Cane, A. Ginouves, S. Marchetti, R. Busca, J. Pouyssegur, E. Berra, P. Hofman & V. Vouret-Craviari (2010). HIF-1alpha mediates the induction of IL-8 and VEGF expression on infection with Afa/Dr diffusely adhering E. coli and promotes EMT-like behaviour, *Cell Microbiol,* Vol.12, No.5, pp.640-53, ISSN 1462-5822

Y. J. Jung, J. S. Isaacs, S. Lee, J. Trepel & L. Neckers (2003). IL-1beta-mediated up-regulation of HIF-1alpha via an NFkappaB/COX-2 pathway identifies HIF-1 as a critical link between inflammation and oncogenesis, *FASEB J,* Vol.17, No.14, pp.2115-7, ISSN 1530-6860

C. Peyssonnaux, A. T. Boutin, A. S. Zinkernagel, V. Datta, V. Nizet & R. S. Johnson (2008). Critical role of HIF-1alpha in keratinocyte defense against bacterial infection, *J Invest Dermatol,* Vol.128, No.8, pp.1964-8, ISSN 1523-1747

J. Zhou, T. Schmid & B. Brune (2003). Tumor necrosis factor-alpha causes accumulation of a ubiquitinated form of hypoxia inducible factor-1alpha through a nuclear factor-kappaB-dependent pathway, *Mol Biol Cell,* Vol.14, No.6, pp.2216-25, ISSN 1059-1524

M. H. Yang, M. Z. Wu, S. H. Chiou, P. M. Chen, S. Y. Chang, C. J. Liu, S. C. Teng & K. J. Wu (2008). Direct regulation of TWIST by HIF-1alpha promotes metastasis, *Nat Cell Biol,* Vol.10, No.3, pp.295-305, ISSN 1476-4679

Q. Li & I. M. Verma (2002). NF-kappaB regulation in the immune system, *Nat Rev Immunol,* Vol.2, No.10, pp.725-34, ISSN 1474-1733

C. Min, S. F. Eddy, D. H. Sherr & G. E. Sonenshein (2008). NF-kappaB and epithelial to mesenchymal transition of cancer, *J Cell Biochem,* Vol.104, No.3, pp.733-44, ISSN 1097-4644

M. Katoh (2009). Integrative genomic analyses of ZEB2: Transcriptional regulation of ZEB2 based on SMADs, ETS1, HIF1alpha, POU/OCT, and NF-kappaB, *Int J Oncol,* Vol.34, No.6, pp.1737-42, ISSN 1019-6439

D. Sosic, J. A. Richardson, K. Yu, D. M. Ornitz & E. N. Olson (2003). Twist regulates cytokine gene expression through a negative feedback loop that represses NF-kappaB activity, *Cell,* Vol.112, No.2, pp.169-80, ISSN 0092-8674

A. J. Pantuck, J. An, H. Liu & M. B. Rettig (2010). NF-kappaB-dependent plasticity of the epithelial to mesenchymal transition induced by Von Hippel-Lindau inactivation in renal cell carcinomas, *Cancer Res,* Vol.70, No.2, pp.752-61, ISSN 1538-7445

A. Lilienbaum, M. Duc Dodon, C. Alexandre, L. Gazzolo & D. Paulin (1990). Effect of human T-cell leukemia virus type I tax protein on activation of the human vimentin gene, *J Virol,* Vol.64, No.1, pp.256-63, ISSN 0022-538X

H. L. Chua, P. Bhat-Nakshatri, S. E. Clare, A. Morimiya, S. Badve & H. Nakshatri (2007). NF-kappaB represses E-cadherin expression and enhances epithelial to mesenchymal transition of mammary epithelial cells: potential involvement of ZEB-1 and ZEB-2, *Oncogene,* Vol.26, No.5, pp.711-24, ISSN 0950-9232

B. P. Himelstein, E. J. Lee, H. Sato, M. Seiki & R. J. Muschel (1997). Transcriptional activation of the matrix metalloproteinase-9 gene in an H-ras and v-myc transformed rat embryo cell line, *Oncogene,* Vol.14, No.16, pp.1995-8, ISSN 0950-9232

T. Yoshizaki, H. Sato & M. Furukawa (2002). Recent advances in the regulation of matrix metalloproteinase 2 activation: from basic research to clinical implication (Review), *Oncol Rep,* Vol.9, No.3, pp.607-11, ISSN 1021-335X

B. P. Lewis, C. B. Burge & D. P. Bartel (2005). Conserved seed pairing, often flanked by adenosines, indicates that thousands of human genes are microRNA targets, *Cell,* Vol.120, No.1, pp.15-20, ISSN 0092-8674

C. P. Bracken, P. A. Gregory, N. Kolesnikoff, A. G. Bert, J. Wang, M. F. Shannon & G. J. Goodall (2008). A double-negative feedback loop between ZEB1-SIP1 and the microRNA-200 family regulates epithelial-mesenchymal transition, *Cancer Res,* Vol.68, No.19, pp.7846-54, ISSN 1538-7445

P. A. Gregory, A. G. Bert, E. L. Paterson, S. C. Barry, A. Tsykin, G. Farshid, M. A. Vadas, Y. Khew-Goodall & G. J. Goodall (2008). The miR-200 family and miR-205 regulate epithelial to mesenchymal transition by targeting ZEB1 and SIP1, *Nat Cell Biol,* Vol.10, No.5, pp.593-601, ISSN 1476-4679

M. Korpal, E. S. Lee, G. Hu & Y. Kang (2008). The miR-200 family inhibits epithelial-mesenchymal transition and cancer cell migration by direct targeting of E-cadherin transcriptional repressors ZEB1 and ZEB2, *J Biol Chem,* Vol.283, No.22, pp.14910-4, ISSN 0021-9258

S. M. Park, A. B. Gaur, E. Lengyel & M. E. Peter (2008). The miR-200 family determines the epithelial phenotype of cancer cells by targeting the E-cadherin repressors ZEB1 and ZEB2, *Genes Dev,* Vol.22, No.7, pp.894-907, ISSN 0890-9369

J. Zavadil, M. Narasimhan, M. Blumenberg & R. J. Schneider (2007). Transforming growth factor-beta and microRNA:mRNA regulatory networks in epithelial plasticity, *Cells Tissues Organs,* Vol.185, No.1-3, pp.157-61, ISSN 1422-6421

C. A. Janeway, Jr. (1989). Approaching the asymptote? Evolution and revolution in immunology, *Cold Spring Harb Symp Quant Biol,* Vol.54 Pt 1, pp.1-13, ISSN 0091-7451

A. Poltorak, X. He, I. Smirnova, M. Y. Liu, C. Van Huffel, X. Du, D. Birdwell, E. Alejos, M. Silva, C. Galanos, M. Freudenberg, P. Ricciardi-Castagnoli, B. Layton & B. Beutler (1998). Defective LPS signaling in C3H/HeJ and C57BL/10ScCr mice: mutations in Tlr4 gene, *Science,* Vol.282, No.5396, pp.2085-8, ISSN 0036-8075

T. Kawai & S. Akira (2010). The role of pattern-recognition receptors in innate immunity: update on Toll-like receptors, *Nat Immunol,* Vol.11, No.5, pp.373-84, ISSN 1529-2916

J. H. Fritz, R. L. Ferrero, D. J. Philpott & S. E. Girardin (2006). Nod-like proteins in immunity, inflammation and disease, *Nat Immunol,* Vol.7, No.12, pp.1250-7, ISSN 1529-2908

A. Bouchon, J. Dietrich & M. Colonna (2000). Cutting edge: inflammatory responses can be triggered by TREM-1, a novel receptor expressed on neutrophils and monocytes, *J Immunol,* Vol.164, No.10, pp.4991-5, ISSN 0022-1767

P. R. Crocker (2005). Siglecs in innate immunity, *Curr Opin Pharmacol,* Vol.5, No.4, pp.431-7, ISSN 1471-4892

J. Klesney-Tait, I. R. Turnbull & M. Colonna (2006). The TREM receptor family and signal integration, *Nat Immunol,* Vol.7, No.12, pp.1266-73, ISSN 1529-2908

M. J. Robinson, D. Sancho, E. C. Slack, S. LeibundGut-Landmann & C. Reis e Sousa (2006). Myeloid C-type lectins in innate immunity, *Nat Immunol,* Vol.7, No.12, pp.1258-65, ISSN 1529-2908

R. E. Ley, D. A. Peterson & J. I. Gordon (2006). Ecological and evolutionary forces shaping microbial diversity in the human intestine, *Cell,* Vol.124, No.4, pp.837-48, ISSN 0092-8674

H. Inagaki, T. Suzuki, K. Nomoto & Y. Yoshikai (1996). Increased susceptibility to primary infection with Listeria monocytogenes in germfree mice may be due to lack of accumulation of L-selectin+ CD44+ T cells in sites of inflammation, *Infect Immun,* Vol.64, No.8, pp.3280-7, ISSN 0019-9567

J. L. Round & S. K. Mazmanian (2009). The gut microbiota shapes intestinal immune responses during health and disease, *Nat Rev Immunol,* Vol.9, No.5, pp.313-23, ISSN 1474-1741

L. Zhao, R. Yang, L. Cheng, M. Wang, Y. Jiang & S. Wang (2010). LPS-Induced Epithelial-Mesenchymal Transition of Intrahepatic Biliary Epithelial Cells, *J Surg Res,* ISSN 1095-8673

M. R. Amieva & E. M. El-Omar (2008). Host-bacterial interactions in Helicobacter pylori infection, *Gastroenterology,* Vol.134, No.1, pp.306-23, ISSN 1528-0012

E. Papini, B. Satin, N. Norais, M. de Bernard, J. L. Telford, R. Rappuoli & C. Montecucco (1998). Selective increase of the permeability of polarized epithelial cell monolayers by Helicobacter pylori vacuolating toxin, *J Clin Invest,* Vol.102, No.4, pp.813-20, ISSN 0021-9738

M. R. Amieva, R. Vogelmann, A. Covacci, L. S. Tompkins, W. J. Nelson & S. Falkow (2003). Disruption of the epithelial apical-junctional complex by Helicobacter pylori CagA, *Science,* Vol.300, No.5624, pp.1430-4, ISSN 1095-9203

N. Murata-Kamiya, Y. Kurashima, Y. Teishikata, Y. Yamahashi, Y. Saito, H. Higashi, H. Aburatani, T. Akiyama, R. M. Peek, Jr., T. Azuma & M. Hatakeyama (2007). Helicobacter pylori CagA interacts with E-cadherin and deregulates the beta-catenin signal that promotes intestinal transdifferentiation in gastric epithelial cells, *Oncogene,* Vol.26, No.32, pp.4617-26, ISSN 0950-9232

Y. Yin, A. M. Grabowska, P. A. Clarke, E. Whelband, K. Robinson, R. H. Argent, A. Tobias, R. Kumari, J. C. Atherton & S. A. Watson (2010). Helicobacter pylori potentiates epithelial:mesenchymal transition in gastric cancer: links to soluble HB-EGF, gastrin and matrix metalloproteinase-7, *Gut,* Vol.59, No.8, pp.1037-45, ISSN 1468-3288

S. Brandt, T. Kwok, R. Hartig, W. Konig & S. Backert (2005). NF-kappaB activation and potentiation of proinflammatory responses by the Helicobacter pylori CagA protein, *Proc Natl Acad Sci U S A,* Vol.102, No.26, pp.9300-5, ISSN 0027-8424

J. H. Park, T. Y. Kim, H. S. Jong, Y. S. Chun, J. W. Park, C. T. Lee, H. C. Jung, N. K. Kim & Y. J. Bang (2003). Gastric epithelial reactive oxygen species prevent normoxic degradation of hypoxia-inducible factor-1alpha in gastric cancer cells, *Clin Cancer Res,* Vol.9, No.1, pp.433-40, ISSN 1078-0432

D. Bagchi, G. Bhattacharya & S. J. Stohs (1996). Production of reactive oxygen species by gastric cells in association with Helicobacter pylori, *Free Radic Res,* Vol.24, No.6, pp.439-50, ISSN 1071-5762

J. B. Kaper, J. P. Nataro & H. L. Mobley (2004). Pathogenic Escherichia coli, *Nat Rev Microbiol,* Vol.2, No.2, pp.123-40, ISSN 1740-1526

A. L. Servin (2005). Pathogenesis of Afa/Dr diffusely adhering Escherichia coli, *Clin Microbiol Rev,* Vol.18, No.2, pp.264-92, ISSN 0893-8512

I. M. Meraz, K. Arikawa, H. Nakamura, J. Ogasawara, A. Hase & Y. Nishikawa (2007). Association of IL-8-inducing strains of diffusely adherent Escherichia coli with sporadic diarrheal patients with less than 5 years of age, *Braz J Infect Dis,* Vol.11, No.1, pp.44-9, ISSN 1413-8670

M. Vargas, J. Gascon, F. Gallardo, M. T. Jimenez De Anta & J. Vila (1998). Prevalence of diarrheagenic Escherichia coli strains detected by PCR in patients with travelers' diarrhea, *Clin Microbiol Infect,* Vol.4, No.12, pp.682-688, ISSN 1469-0691

C. N. Berger, O. Billker, T. F. Meyer, A. L. Servin & I. Kansau (2004). Differential recognition of members of the carcinoembryonic antigen family by Afa/Dr adhesins of diffusely adhering Escherichia coli (Afa/Dr DAEC), *Mol Microbiol,* Vol.52, No.4, pp.963-83, ISSN 0950-382X

F. Betis, P. Brest, V. Hofman, J. Guignot, M. F. Bernet-Camard, B. Rossi, A. Servin & P. Hofman (2003a). The Afa/Dr adhesins of diffusely adhering Escherichia coli stimulate interleukin-8 secretion, activate mitogen-activated protein kinases, and promote polymorphonuclear transepithelial migration in T84 polarized epithelial cells, *Infect Immun,* Vol.71, No.3, pp.1068-74, ISSN 0019-9567

F. Betis, P. Brest, V. Hofman, J. Guignot, I. Kansau, B. Rossi, A. Servin & P. Hofman (2003b). Afa/Dr diffusely adhering Escherichia coli infection in T84 cell monolayers induces increased neutrophil transepithelial migration, which in turn promotes cytokine-dependent upregulation of decay-accelerating factor (CD55), the receptor for Afa/Dr adhesins, *Infect Immun,* Vol.71, No.4, pp.1774-83, ISSN 0019-9567

G. Cane, V. L. Moal, G. Pages, A. L. Servin, P. Hofman & V. Vouret-Craviari (2007). Up-regulation of intestinal vascular endothelial growth factor by Afa/Dr diffusely adhering Escherichia coli, *PLoS One,* Vol.2, No.12, pp.e1359, ISSN 1932-6203

V. A. Rathinam & K. A. Fitzgerald (2011). Innate immune sensing of DNA viruses, *Virology,* Vol.411, No.2, pp.153-62, ISSN 1096-0341

M.-R. Chen (2011). Epstein-Barr virus, the immune system, and associated diseases, *Front. Microbio.,* Vol.2:5, ISSN

R. G. Caldwell, J. B. Wilson, S. J. Anderson & R. Longnecker (1998). Epstein-Barr virus LMP2A drives B cell development and survival in the absence of normal B cell receptor signals, *Immunity,* Vol.9, No.3, pp.405-11, ISSN 1074-7613

O. Gires, U. Zimber-Strobl, R. Gonnella, M. Ueffing, G. Marschall, R. Zeidler, D. Pich & W. Hammerschmidt (1997). Latent membrane protein 1 of Epstein-Barr virus mimics a constitutively active receptor molecule, *EMBO J,* Vol.16, No.20, pp.6131-40, ISSN 0261-4189

T. Horikawa, J. Yang, S. Kondo, T. Yoshizaki, I. Joab, M. Furukawa & J. S. Pagano (2007). Twist and epithelial-mesenchymal transition are induced by the EBV oncoprotein latent membrane protein 1 and are associated with metastatic nasopharyngeal carcinoma, *Cancer Res,* Vol.67, No.5, pp.1970-8, ISSN 0008-5472

T. Horikawa, T. Yoshizaki, S. Kondo, M. Furukawa, Y. Kaizaki & J. S. Pagano (2011). Epstein-Barr Virus latent membrane protein 1 induces Snail and epithelial-mesenchymal transition in metastatic nasopharyngeal carcinoma, *Br J Cancer,* Vol.104, No.7, pp.1160-7, ISSN 1532-1827

Q. L. Kong, L. J. Hu, J. Y. Cao, Y. J. Huang, L. H. Xu, Y. Liang, D. Xiong, S. Guan, B. H. Guo, H. Q. Mai, Q. Y. Chen, X. Zhang, M. Z. Li, J. Y. Shao, C. N. Qian, Y. F. Xia, L. B.

Song, Y. X. Zeng & M. S. Zeng (2010). Epstein-Barr virus-encoded LMP2A induces an epithelial-mesenchymal transition and increases the number of side population stem-like cancer cells in nasopharyngeal carcinoma, *PLoS Pathog,* Vol.6, No.6, pp.e1000940, ISSN 1553-7374

A. Shinozaki, T. Sakatani, T. Ushiku, R. Hino, M. Isogai, S. Ishikawa, H. Uozaki, K. Takada & M. Fukayama (2010). Downregulation of microRNA-200 in EBV-associated gastric carcinoma, *Cancer Res,* Vol.70, No.11, pp.4719-27, ISSN 1538-7445

A. P. Malizia, N. Lacey, D. Walls, J. J. Egan & P. P. Doran (2009). CUX1/Wnt signaling regulates epithelial mesenchymal transition in EBV infected epithelial cells, *Exp Cell Res,* Vol.315, No.11, pp.1819-31, ISSN 1090-2422

M. D. Sides, R. C. Klingsberg, B. Shan, K. A. Gordon, H. T. Nguyen, Z. Lin, T. Takahashi, E. K. Flemington & J. A. Lasky (2011). The Epstein-Barr virus latent membrane protein 1 and transforming growth factor--beta1 synergistically induce epithelial--mesenchymal transition in lung epithelial cells, *Am J Respir Cell Mol Biol,* Vol.44, No.6, pp.852-62, ISSN 1535-4989

S. Z. Yang, L. D. Zhang, Y. Zhang, Y. Xiong, Y. J. Zhang, H. L. Li, X. W. Li & J. H. Dong (2009). HBx protein induces EMT through c-Src activation in SMMC-7721 hepatoma cell line, *Biochem Biophys Res Commun,* Vol.382, No.3, pp.555-60, ISSN 1090-2104

N. Delhem, A. Sabile, R. Gajardo, P. Podevin, A. Abadie, M. A. Blaton, D. Kremsdorf, L. Beretta & C. Brechot (2001). Activation of the interferon-inducible protein kinase PKR by hepatocellular carcinoma derived-hepatitis C virus core protein, *Oncogene,* Vol.20, No.41, pp.5836-45, ISSN 0950-9232

M. M. Lai & C. F. Ware (2000). Hepatitis C virus core protein: possible roles in viral pathogenesis, *Curr Top Microbiol Immunol,* Vol.242, pp.117-34, ISSN 0070-217X

N. Zhu, A. Khoshnan, R. Schneider, M. Matsumoto, G. Dennert, C. Ware & M. M. Lai (1998). Hepatitis C virus core protein binds to the cytoplasmic domain of tumor necrosis factor (TNF) receptor 1 and enhances TNF-induced apoptosis, *J Virol,* Vol.72, No.5, pp.3691-7, ISSN 0022-538X

N. Pavio, S. Battaglia, D. Boucreux, B. Arnulf, R. Sobesky, O. Hermine & C. Brechot (2005). Hepatitis C virus core variants isolated from liver tumor but not from adjacent non-tumor tissue interact with Smad3 and inhibit the TGF-beta pathway, *Oncogene,* Vol.24, No.40, pp.6119-32, ISSN 0950-9232

S. Battaglia, N. Benzoubir, S. Nobilet, P. Charneau, D. Samuel, A. L. Zignego, A. Atfi, C. Brechot & M. F. Bourgeade (2009). Liver cancer-derived hepatitis C virus core proteins shift TGF-beta responses from tumor suppression to epithelial-mesenchymal transition, *PLoS One,* Vol.4, No.2, pp.e4355, ISSN 1932-6203

T. Li, D. Li, L. Cheng, H. Wu, Z. Gao, Z. Liu, W. Jiang, Y. H. Gao, F. Tian, L. Zhao & S. Wang (2010). Epithelial-mesenchymal transition induced by hepatitis C virus core protein in cholangiocarcinoma, *Ann Surg Oncol,* Vol.17, No.7, pp.1937-44, ISSN 1534-4681

P. M. Hofman (2010). Pathobiology of the neutrophil-intestinal epithelial cell interaction: role in carcinogenesis, *World J Gastroenterol,* Vol.16, No.46, pp.5790-800, ISSN 1007-9327

4

Cytokeratin 7 and 20

Agnieszka Jasik
National Veterinary Research Institute
Poland

1. Introduction

Intermediate filaments (IFs) are the most stable components in the cells, and are involved in many important physiological functions, including distribution of organelles, signal transduction, cell polarity and gene regulation. (Iwatsuki & Suda, 2010).

Cytokeratins (CK or CKs) are the largest complex group of IF proteins. These are proteins, that are crucial in the development and differentiation of epithelial cells, as well as essential for normal tissue structure and function. The first keratin protein nomenclature was published by Moll et al. (1982) and it has been repeatedly updated in recent years (Schweizer et al., 2006). Based on the results of ongoing research in human and other vertebrates, Szeverenyi et al. (2008) published a comprehensive catalogue of the human keratins, their amino acid sequence, the nucleotide sequence of the keratin genes in humans, as well as the same data of the orthologue keratins and keratin genes in various vertebrate species. Based on their molecular weights and isoelectric points CKs were catalogued and divided into two groups: type I and type II cytokeratins. The type I cytokeratins consist of acidic, low molecular weight (40-56.5 kDa) proteins including cytokeratins K9-K28 and hair keratins K31-K40. The type II cytokeratins consist of basic, high molecular weight (52-67 kDa) proteins including cytokeratins K1-K8, cytokeratins K71-K80 and hair keratins K81-K86 (Bragulla & Homberger, 2009; Iwatsuki & Suda, 2010; Moll et al., 2008; Schweizer et al., 2006). Cytokeratins are relatively resistant to degradation and show highly specific phenotypic expression depending on the type and differentiation of the epithelial cells. Hence, the different types of epithelia have specific for them pattern of keratin expression.

Based on biochemical and immunohistochemical studies, it was possible to explain and define the epithelial tissue-specific distribution of CKs but also to conclude that tumors arising from a given epithelium generally preserved this pattern of CK expression despite malignant transformation. Moreover, the cytokeratin expression patterns in a given type of tumor appear to be identical in primary tumors and their metastases, independent from the specific location and size (Lam et al., 2001; Moll et al., 1982). Therefore, antibodies against various cytokeratins are important in the accurate identification and classification of different types of carcinomas, whose origin is uncertain by routine light microscopy. In this context, the diverse expression patterns of CK7 and CK 20 among epithelial tumors have been proposed to help discriminating primary from metastatic carcinoma of various origins (Duval et al., 2000; Nikitakis et al., 2004; Wauters et al., 1995). Based on the differential staining patterns for cytokeratins reported in the literature, in the following chapter, we focused on evaluation of utility of cytokeratins 7 and 20 both in differential diagnosis of tumors and identification of the primary site of tumor origin.

2. Characterization and distribution of cytokeratins 7 and 20 in tissues

2.1 Cytokeratin 7

Cytokeratin 7 (CK7) is a polypeptide with molecular weight 54 kDa and an isoelectric point at pH 6.0. (Bragulla & Homberger, 2009; Moll et al., 1982; Schweizer et al., 2006). This protein is encoded by the KRT7 gene, located on chromosome 12q13.13 (Bragulla & Homberger, 2009, Schweizer et al., 2006). In normal tissues, this basic (type II) keratin is found to be distributed in a wide variety of simple epithelia: in organs associated with the gastrointestinal tract (including only the gallbladder, hepatic ducts and pancreatic ducts), female genital tract (the ovary, endometrium, fallopian tube and cervix), breast, urinary tract (the cells of the renal tubule and collecting ducts of the kidney, as well as in the cells of the transitional epithelium of the mucosa of the renal pelvis, ureter and bladder), and respiratory tract (the sinonasal mucosa, trachea and lung) (Iwatsuki & Suda, 2010; Moll et al., 1982, 2008). Cytokeratin 7 is found in epithelial cells of fetal stomach, whereas in normal gastrointestinal epithelium is undetectable (Tatsumi et al., 2005). It is also one of the several cytokeratins, which are expressed in the developing teeth of human (in the developing stratified enamel organ) (Bragulla & Homberger, 2009). In endometrium, CK7 expression is high in secretory phase but low in the proliferative phase of the estrous cycle. Cytokeratin 7 is also expressed in the epithelial cells of the nail bed epidermis and in mesothelium and endothelial cells. Moreover, CK7 has been shown to be expressed to a different degree in the various epithelial salivary gland elements; more specifically, immunohistochemicaly the luminal cells of the salivary ducts are strongly positive for CK7, while the acinar, basal, and myoepithelial cells stain with less intensity (Nikitakis et al., 2004). Cytokeratin 7 was undetectable in hepatocytes, proximal and distal tubules of the kidney, and squamous cell epithelia.

2.2 Cytokeratin 20

Cytokeratin 20 (CK20) is a newly described polypeptide with molecular weight 48.5 kDa and an isoelectric point at pH 5.66 (Bragulla & Homberger, 2009; Moll et al., 1993; Schweizer et al., 2006). This protein is encoded by the KRT20 gene, located on chromosome 17q21.2 (Bragulla & Homberger, 2009, Schweizer et al., 2006). CK20 was originally identified as protein "IT" in cytoskeletal extracts of intestinal epithelia. In normal human tissues this acidic (type I) keratin is found in more complex epithelia of the gastrointestinal tract (such as taste buds, gastric foveolar cells and intestinal epithelium), urothelial umbrella cells, squamous epithelia from any site and Merkel cells of the epidermis and hair follicle outer root sheath (Barret et al., 2000; Jovanovic et al., 2002; Moll et al., 2008). In human embryogenesis, it appears in the small intestinal epithelium at embryonic week 8 (Moll et al., 2008). No cytokeratin 20 expression was identified in mesothelium (Tot, 2002), sinonasal epithelia (Franchi et al., 2004) and any salivary gland epithelial elements (Nikitakis et al., 2004).

3. Application of cytokeratins 7 and 20 in diagnostic pathology

3.1 Expression of CK7 in primary tumors and their metastases

The frequency of CK 7 expression is summarized in Figure 1. Generally positive immunohistochemical cytokeratin 7 expression has been identified in carcinomas of the breast, lung, endometrium and ovaries. Moreover, primary tumors of the sinonasal tract, thyroid gland, salivary gland, biliary and urinary tract stain strongly positive for CK7.

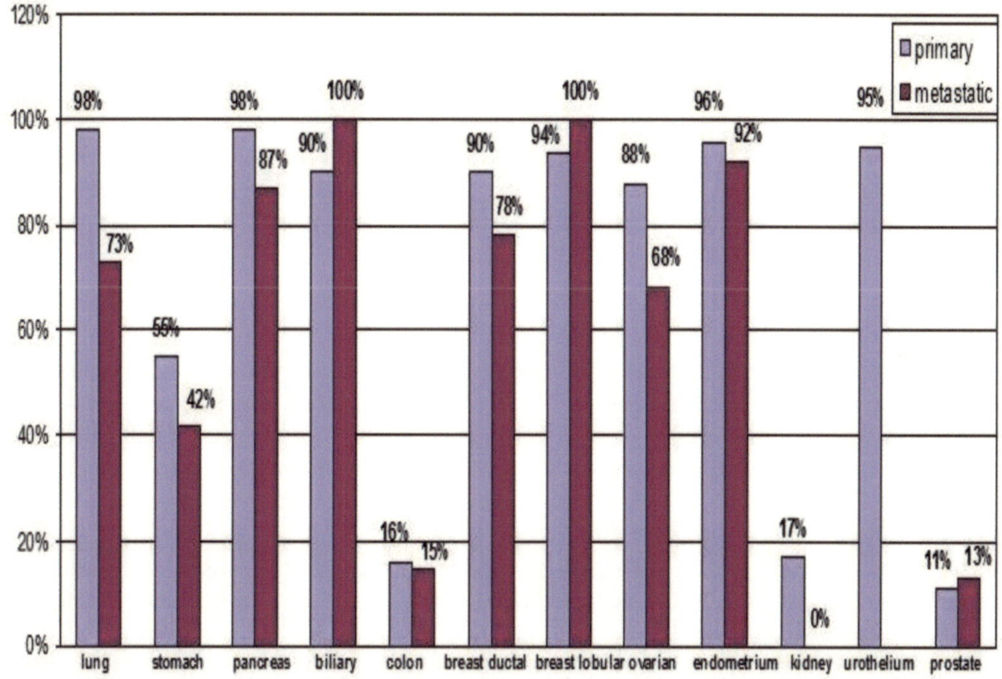

Fig. 1. Percentage of positive expression of CK7 in primary and metastatic adenocarcinomas (based on Tot, 2002)

Even some primary brain neoplasms, like choroid plexus tumors, as well as malignant mesotheliomas and synovial sarcomas are CK7+. Taking to account the different histological subtypes of cancer, CK7 positivity has been reported in 100% of cases of papillary thyroid carcinoma (86/86), follicular thyroid carcinoma (19/19) and medullary thyroid carcinoma (13/13) (Lam et al., 2001) as well as mucinous (6/6), nonmucinous (4/4) and mixed (6/6) bronchioloalveolar adenocarcinoma (Chu et al., 2000; Simsir et al., 2004).

The same percentage of positive immunostaining for CK7 was detected in seven histologic types of salivary gland carcinoma, including mucoepidermoid, adenoid cystic, polymorphous low grade, salivary duct, acinic cell, clear cell and basal cell (Nikitakis et al., 2004). Poorly differentiated and anaplastic thyroid carcinomas expressed CK7, but the number of immunoreactive cells was smaller than those in well-diferentiated carcinomas. Similarly the percentage of CK7 positive cases of urothelial carcinoma was lower in high-grade tumors infiltrating the surrounding tissues (67%), than in low-grade urothelial carcinoma (100%) (Bassily et al., 2000). This may be due to the loss of cytokeratin expression during tumor progression into high-grade lesion.

It is also worth noting that distribution of cytokeratin 7 staining varied among different histological types of some tumors, which may be useful in their discrimination. An example of this is the report by Nikitakis et al. (2004) on salivary gland tumors, describing focal staining of CK7 in adenoid cystic carcinoma compared to the universally diffuse pattern in polymorphous low-grade adenocarcinoma. Also, there was a report of strong cytoplasmic and membrane CK7 staining in chromophobe variant of renal cell carcinoma distinguishing it from benign oncocytomas showing focal weak-to-moderate CK7 cytoplasmic staining (Campbell & Herrington, 2001). Among soft tissue sarcomas CK7 expression has been found in a small proportion of liposarcomas (7%), gastrointestinal stromal tumors (12%) and epithelioid (25%) (Humble et al., 2003) and synovial sarcomas. Other sarcomas, including malignant fibrous histocytoma, leiomyosarcoma, angiosarcoma, malignant peripheral nerve sheath tumor, desmoids tumor, rhabdomyosarcoma and primitive neuroectodermal tumor were negative for CK7 (Campbell & Herrington, 2001). Prostate adenocarcinomas, hepatocellular carcinomas and most of gastric carcinomas also have been negative for keratin 7, despite of small proportion of these tumor cases showing CK7 positive expression (Bassily et al., 2000; Chu et al., 2000; Sawan, 2009).

Nevertheless, the lack of immunoreactivity in colorectal adenocarcinomas is the main point of diagnostic utility of this keratin in differentiation adenocarcinoma metastases in context of their possible primary tumor. Eighty-eight percent of metastases from colorectal adenocarcinoma to the lung, liver, lymph nodes, chin, small bowel, peritoneum and bone were negative for CK7 (Kummar et al., 2002). Respectively, 62.5 % (Rekhi et al., 2008) and 76.4% (Wauters et al., 1995) of colorectal adenocarcinoma metastases to the ovary were also negative for CK7. Despite the lack of expression of cytokeratin 7, some cases of colorectal adenocarcinoma show positive immunoreactivity for CK7. This positive rate for CK7 is 0-16% in primary tumors, and 8.3-19% in metastatic cancers. In contrast, almost 100% and 73% immunoreactivity for CK7 has been detected in primary and metastatic pulmonary adenocarcinomas respectively.

3.2 Expression of CK20 in primary tumors and their metastases

The frequency of CK 20 expression is summarized in Figure 2. CK20 expression is restricted to a few organ systems. Almost all cases of colon carcinoma (91-100%) were positive for CK20, as well as 64-78% of urothelial tumors, 78% of Merkel cell tumors, 50-71% of adenocarcinomas of the stomach, 55% of biliary adenocarcinomas and 44-62% of adenocarcinomas of the pancreas (Chu et al., 2000; Duval et al., 2000; Stopyra et al., 2001; Tot, 2002).

Moreover, high percentage (84%) of sinonasal intestinal-type adenocarcinomas (ITACs) was CK20 positive, which distinguished them from non-ITACs showing lack of immunoreactivity for CK20 (Franchi et al., 2004). Similarly, in the case of renal oncocytomas a high degree of CK20 positive immunoreactivity (80%) can be a useful diagnostic tool to distinguish them from renal cell carcinomas, in which no or weak positive reaction (range 0-7.7%) has been found (Stopyra et al., 2001).

In all of the colorectal lesions high CK20 positivity was found, including 100% in hyperplastic polyps, 95% in serrated adenomas, 90% in conventional adenomas and 92% in adenocarcinomas. Generally, pulmonary adenocarcinomas are negative for CK20 (Campbell & Herrington, 2001; Hatanaka et al., 2011; Kummar et al., 2002). Nevertheless, positive immunoreactivity for CK20 has been detected in 5 (83%) of 6 cases of mucinous and in all (6) cases of mixed bronchioloalveolar carcinoma (Simsir et al., 2004), as well as in 5 (32%) of 16 cases of pulmonary adenocarcinoma with enteric differentiation (Hatanaka et al., 2011). All cases of nonmucinous bronchioloalveolar carcinomas were negative for CK20 (Simsir et al., 2004). For this reason, distinguishing primary pulmonary adenocarcinomas from metastases with strong CK20 expression may be difficult. There are some differences in CK20 expression in ovarian adenocarcinomas. About 67% of ovarian mucinous adenocarcinomas were positive for CK20, while among non-mucinous ovarian tumors 25% (62/246) expressed CK20 (Tot, 2002; Wauters et al., 1995). The lack of reaction, or sporadic focal and weak CK20 immunostaining is detected in salivary gland tumors, except small cell carcinomas, that frequently display diffuse positivity for CK20. Those cases included: 2 (7.7%) of 26 cases of mucoepidermoid carcinoma, 1 (4%) of 25 cases of adenoid cystic carcinoma and 3 (37.5%) of 8 cases of salivary duct carcinoma (Nikitakis et al., 2004), as well as 6 (10%) of 59 cases of prostate adenocarcinoma (Campbell & Herrington, 2001) and 2 (6%) of 30 cases of squmous cell carcinoma of the head and neck (Chu et al., 2000). So far, no cytokeratin 20 expression has been found in soft tissue sarcomas, such as epithelioid sarcoma, malignant fibrous histiocytoma, malignant peripheral nerve sheath tumor, leiomyosarcoma, angiosarcoma, desmoids tumor, rhabdomyosarcoma and primitive neuroectodermal tumor (Campbell & Herrington, 2002). Lack of CK20 reactivity was also reported in all thyroid carcinomas (Lam et al., 2001), thymomas, mesotheliomas (Campbell & Herrington, 2001), and squamous cell carcinomas of the cervix (Chu et al., 2000; Nikitakis et al., 2004).

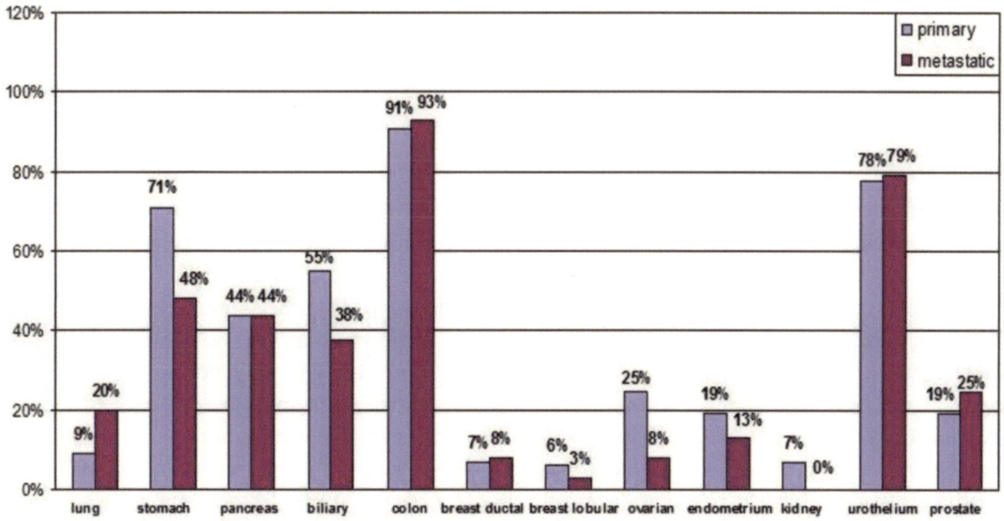

Fig. 2. Percentage of positive expression of CK20 in primary and metastatic adenocarcinomas (based on Tot 2002)

Strong stability of the CK20 expression in colorectal adenocarcinomas (Table 2), that retain during their metastatic progression allows for specific recognition of metastases of this type of tumor. Ninety-two percent of metastases of the colorectal cancers to the lung, liver, lymph nodes and small bowel were positive for CK20 (Tot, 2002; Kummar et al., 2002).

Colorectal adenocarcinomas metastatic to the ovary also showed CK20 positivity in all cases. However, in the latter case, primary mucinous ovarian carcinomas can not be excluded, due to their positive expression of CK20. The fact, that tumors retain expression of CK20 during their metastases, is useful in detection of circulating cancer cell in the peripheral blood, using reverse transcriptase (RT)-PCR analysis. It is a very helpful method to detect metastases at a very early stage of disease, especially in case of colorectal carcinoma, gastric and pancreatic adenocarcinoma as well as lung carcinoma (Moll et al., 2008; Wang et al., 2006). The same method is used in early detection of bladder cancer in voided urine (Pu et al., 2007).

3.3 CK7/CK20 phenotype in primary tumors and metastases

Among epithelial tumors approximately 80% are malignant (Chu et al., 2000).

Metastatic tumors from an uknown primary site are a common clinical problem, that leads to extensive and costly clinical and radiological examinations, sometimes with disappointing results. A proper diagnosis of the primary site is important for therapeutic decision-making and prognosis of particular tumor types.

Possibility of identifying the primary tumors in cases of unclear metastases is significantly increased when CK7 is used in combination with CK20, since many carcinomas exhibit characteristic CK7/CK20 phenotypes. For the determination of these phenotypes several monoclonal antibodies against CK7 and CK20 are used (Upasani et al., 2004). Most commonly used antibodies, their dilutions and the antigen retrieval methods are presented in Table 1. For comparison, the distribution of reported CK7/CK20 phenotype of different types of tumor in the reviewed literature is presented in Table 2. Differences between a specific type of tumor and its CK7/CK20 phenotype found in the collected literature make it difficult to compare the results. Therefore, the data presented in the table should be considered as a collection of information published so far.

The majority of the tumor cases from the gastrointestinal and genitourinary tracts, which have been described so far show CK7+/CK20+ phenotype. This phenotype is also very specific for mucinous and mixed bronchioloalveolar adenocarcionomas (BACs) and differs from typical CK7+/CK20- phenotype of conventional pulmonary adenocarcinoma. This immunohistochemical staining is crucial for distinguishing mucinous and mixed BACs from metastatic adenocarcinomas involving the lungs. Nevertheless, distinction of mucinous BACs from metastatic mucinous adenocarcinomas of gastrointestinal, pancreatic, and ovarian origins can be difficult, due to the same CK7+/CK20+ phenotype. To distinguish prostate carcinoma from urothelial carcinoma CK7+/CK20+ phenotype is helpful for ruling out prostate cancer, as it is extremely rarely (0-2%) present in prostate carcinoma (Bassily et al. 2000). Immunophenotype CK7-/CK20+ is most useful in distinguish primary and metastatic tumors from the colorectal tumors and Merkel cell carcinomas (Saeb-Lima et al., 2008). However, it should be kept in mind, that some of recently described primary pulmonary adenocarcinomas with enteric differentiation (12.5%) express the same phenotype (Hatanaka et al., 2011).

Large number of different type of tumors express different percentage of CK7+/CK20- phenotype (Table 2), that is the most specific for tumors of the lungs, sinonasal tract, salivary gland and thyroid gland (Franchi et al., 2004; Lam et al., 2001; Kummar et al., 2002; Nikitakis et al., 2004). Therefore, it is not possible to differentiate these tumor types, based solely on cytokeratin 7 expression. Knowledge of the CK7/CK20 immunophenotype of tumors in case of distant metastases may be valuable in their definitive diagnosis, especially in the lack of a previous diagnosis of a primary tumor. It can be important in case of metastases of colorectal carcinoma and breast tumors to the skin (Fidler et al., 2007). Tumors of the skin and soft tissue, which have been reported so far, express mainly CK7-/CK20- phenotype, beside Merkel cell carcinomas.

Antibody	Clone	Dilution	Source	Antigen retrieval method
	OV-TL 12/30	1:12.5	Dako	without pretreatment
	OV-TL 12/30	1:50	Dako	0.05% pronase , 37 °C
	OV-TL 12/30	1:60	Dako	0.1% pronase, RT (10 min)
	OV-TL 12/30	1:100	Dako	0.01 M citrate buffer pH 6, microwave (15 min)
	OV-TL 12/30	1:100	Bio Genex	0.1% pronase in Tris-HCl buffer, 37°C (5 min)
Cytokeratin 7	OV-TL 12/30	1:200	Dako	0.01 M citrate buffer pH 6, microwave (5 min)
	OV-TL 12/30	1:800	Bio Genex	0.5% protease XIV 20°C (15 min)
	OV-TL 12/30	1:1900	Dako	proteinase K (ready-to-use), RT (10 min)
	LDS-68	1:32000	Sigma	0.4% pepsin in 0.01 N hydrochloric acid, 37°C (15 min)
Cytokeratin 20	Ks 20.8	1:10	Dako	0.1% pronase in Tris-HCl buffer, 37°C (5 min)
	Ks 20.8	1:10	Dako	without pretreatment
	Ks 20.8	1:50	Dako	boiled in 10 mm citrate buffer pH 6
	Ks 20.8	1:60	Dako	0.1% pronase, RT (10 min)
	Ks 20.8	1:60	Bio Genex	0.5% protease XIV 20°C (15 min)
	Ks 20.8	1:100	Dako	0.01 M citrate buffer pH 6, microwave (15 min)
Cytokeratin 20 (RTU-CK20)	Ks 20.8	ready to use	Novocastra	0.01 M citrate buffer pH 6, microwave (20 min)
Cytokeratin 20 (NCL-CK20)	Ks 20.8	1:1350	Novocastra	proteinase K (ready-to-use), RT (10 min)

Table 1. Monoclonal antibodies against CK7 and CK20, their dilution and the antigen retrieval methods

Organ	Tumor type/subtype	CK7+/ CK20+ (%)	CK7+/ CK 20 - (%)	CK7-/ CK20+ (%)	CK7-/ CK20- (%)
Lungs	mixed BAC	100	0	0	0
	mucinous BAC	83	17	0	0
	nonmucinous BAC	0	100	0	0
	PAED	18.75	68.75	12.5	0
	adenocarcinoma	8-10	84-96	0	0
	carcinoid tumors	0	22	0	78
	small cell carcinoma	0	43	0	57
	squamous cell carcinoma	0	47	0	53
	neuroendocrine carcinoma	0	56	0	44
Sinonasal tract	ITAC	80	8	4	8
	non-ITAC	0	100	0	0
Salivary gland	salivary duct carcinoma	37.5	62.5	0	0
	mucoepidermoid carcinoma	7.7	92.3	0	0
	AdCC	4	96	0	0
	PLGA	0	100	0	0
	ACC	0	100	0	0
	Ca-ex-MT	0	100	0	0
	CCC	0	100	0	0
	BCAC	0	100	0	0
Thyroid gland	papillary carinoma	0	100	0	0
	follicular carcinoma	0	100	0	0
	insular carcinoma	0	60	40	0
	anaplastic carcinoma	0	84	0	16
	medullary carcinoma	0	100	0	0
Thymus	thymoma	0	0	0	100
Pancreas	adenocarcinoma	48-62	30-80	0-7	4-8
Liver	hepatocellular carcinoma	0	9-12.5	9	82-87.5
	neuroendocrine carcinoma	0	56	0	44
Biliary tract	cholangiocarcinoma	24-43	50-76	0	7-13
	gallbladder carcinoma	27	55	0	18
Stomach	gastric adenocarcinoma	13-33	24-25	33-37	10-25
Ovary	mucinous adenocarcinoma	76	14	0	0
	nonmucinous adenocarcinoma	7	93	0	0

Organ	Tumor type/subtype	CK7+/ CK20+ (%)	CK7+/ CK 20 - (%)	CK7-/ CK20+ (%)	CK7-/ CK20- (%)
Uterus	endometrial carcinoma	0	100	0	0
	cervical squamous cell carcinoma	0	87	0	13
Breast	infiltrating ductal carcinoma	0	95	0	5
	infiltrating lobular carcinoma	0	100	0	0
Kidney	renal oncocytoma	60	20	20	0
	renal cell carcinoma	0	11	0	89
Bladder	urothelial adenocarcinoma	61	21	4	14
	transitional cell carcinoma	25	63	4	8
Prostate	adenocarcinoma	0-2	0-9	0-14	81-100
Colon	serrated adenoma	71	4.5	25	0
	hyperplastic polyp	68	0	32	0
	adenocarcinoma	5-8.3	1-2.1	83-100	0-6.3
	conventional adenoma	5	0	85	10
	neuroendocrine carcinoma	0	56	0	44
Mesothelium	malignant mesothelioma	0	65	0	35
Skin and soft tissue	merkel cell carcinoma	0	0	78	12
	epithelioid sarcoma	0	0	0	100
	MPNST	0	0	0	100
	MFH	0	0	0	100
	leiomyosarcoma	0	0	0	100
	angiosarcoma	0	0	0	100
	desmoids tumor	0	0	0	100
	rhabdomyosarcoma	0	0	0	100
	primitive neuroectodermal tumor	0	0	0	100

Abbreviations: BAC, bronchioloalveolar adenocarcinoma; PAED, pulmonary adenocarcinoma with enteric differentiation; ITAC, intestinal-type adenocarcinoma; AdCC, adenoid cystic carcinoma; PLGA, polymorphous low-grade adenocarcinoma; ACC, acinic cell carcinoma; Ca-ex-MT, carcinoma ex mixed tumor; CCC, clear cell carcinoma; BCAC, basal cell adenocarcinoma; MPNST, malignant peripheral nerve sheath tumor; MFH, malignant fibrous histiocytoma.

Table 2. Distribution of CK7/CK20 phenotype in different types of tumors of different organs (based on references: Bassily et al., 2000; Cambell & Harrington, 2001; Chu et al., 2000; Duval et al., 2000; Hatanaka et al., 2011; Humble et al., 2003; Kummar et al., 2002;Lam et al., 2001; Nikitakis et al., 2004; Rekhi et al., 2008; Saeb-Lima et al., 2008; Sawan, 2009; Simsir et al., 2004; Stopyra et al., 2001; Tatsumi et al., 2005; Tot, 2002; Wauter at al., 1995)

4. Conclusion

This chapter shows that the CK7/CK20 phenotype of tumors can be a valuable diagnostic marker in the determination of the primary site of origin of metastatic tumor (Fig. 1, 2, Table 2). Detection of CK7+/CK20- phenotype indicates metastatic carcinoma, most often from the lungs, salivary gland or breast in bone, ovaries, liver, colon and even in bone marrow. The CK7-/CK20+ phenotype indicates metastatic carcinoma, usually from the colorectal region mainly in lungs and ovaries. Whereas, the CK7-/CK20- phenotype indicates metastatic carcinoma often from the prostate, mainly in bone. However, the different CK7/CK20 immunophenotypes do not show 100% specificity and sensitivity for any tumor. Therefore, CK7 and CK20 should be used as a part of an immunohistochemical panel of antibodies. Despite the fact, that the data presented in this chapter come from reports from recent years, further studies involving cases of tumors with clearly identified primary location, tumor type and subtype are necessary to confirm these results and to extend CK phenotyping to rare tumor types. Moreover, further studies are needed for evaluation of RT-PCR for CK20 mRNA in serum, blood, urine for the identification of tumor cells. Due to the relatively widespread expression of cytokeratin 7 in epithelial cells of various organs, further research related to the gene KTR7 (Pujal et al., 2009) could be useful in therapeutic strategies for epithelial neoplasms.

5. Acknowledgment

I am grateful to Dr Anna Kycko for her help in correcting the English language.

6. References

Barrett, A.W.; Cort, E.M.; Patel, P. & Berkovitz, B.K.B. (2000). An immunohistochemical study of cytokeratin 20 in human and mammalian oral epithelium. *Archives of Oral Biology*, Vol.45, No.10, pp.879-887, ISSN 0003-9969

Bassily, N.H.; Vallorosi, Ch.J.; Akdas, G.; Montie, J.E. & Rubin, M.A. (2000). Coordinate expression of cytokeratins 7 and 20 in prostate adenocarcinoma and bladder urothelial carcinoma. *American Journal of Clinical Pathology*, Vol.113, No.3, pp.383-388, ISSN 0002-9173

Bragulla, H.H. & Homberger, D.G. (2009). Structure and functions of keratin proteins in simple, stratified, keratinized and cornified epithelia. *Journal of Anatomy*, Vol.214, No.4, pp.516-559, ISSN 0021-8782

Campbell, F. & Herrington, C.S. (2001). Application of cytokeratin 7 and 20 immunohistochemistry to diagnostic pathology. *Current Diagnostic Pathology*, Vol.7, No.2, pp.113-122, ISSN 0968-6053

Chu, P.; Wu, E. & Weiss, L.M. (2000). Cytokeratin 7 and cytokeratin 20 expression in epithelial neoplasms: A survey of 435 cases. *Modern Pathology*, Vol.13, No.9, pp.962-972, ISSN 0893-3952

Duval, J.V.; Savas, L. & Banner, B.F. (2000). Expression of cytokeratins 7 and 20 in carcinomas of the extrahepatic biliary tract, pancreas, and gallbladder. *Archives of Pathology & Laboratory Medicine*, Vol.124, No.8, pp.1196-1200, ISSN 0003-9985

Fiddler, S.; Kaj, J.; Płochocki, M.; Filipczyk-Cisarż, E. & Ziemba, B. (2007). Upper limb amputation in the course of skin metastases of rectal cancer. *Onkologia w Praktyce Klinicznej*, Vol. 3, No.5, pp.259-262, ISSN 1734-3542

Franchi, A.; Massi, D.; Plomba, A.; Biancalani, M. & Santucci, M. (2004). CDX-2, cytokeratin 7 and cytokeratin 20 immunohistochemical expression in the differentia diagnosis of primary adenocarcinomas of the sinonasal tract. *Virchows Arch*, Vol.445, No.1, pp.63-67, ISSN 1432-2307

Hatanaka, K.; Tsuta, K.; Watanabe, K.; Sugino, K. & Uekusa, T. (2011). Primary pulmonary adenocarcinoma with enteric differentiation resembling metastatic colorectal carcinoma: A report of the second case negative for cytokeratin 7. *PathologyResearch and Practice*, Vol.207, No.3, pp.188-191, ISSN 0344-0338

Humble, S.D.; Prieto, V.G. & Horenstein, M.G. (2003). Cytokeratin 7 and 20 expression in epithelioid sarcoma. *Journal of Cutaneous Pathology*, Vol.30, No.4, pp.242-246, ISSN 0303-6987

Iwatsuki, H. & Suda, M. (2010). Seven kinds of intermediate filament networks in the cytoplasm of polarized cells: structure and function. *Acta Histochemica et Cytochemica*, Vol.43, No.2, pp.19-31, ISSN 0044-5991

Jovanovic, I.; Tzardi, M.; Mouzas, I.A.; Micev, M.; Pesko, P.; Milosavljevic, T.; Zois, M.; Sganzos, M.; Delides, G. & Kanavaros, P. (2002). Changing pattern of cytokeratin 7 and 20 expression from normal epithelium to intestinal metaplasia of the gastric mucosa and gastroesophageal junction. *Histology and Histopathology*, Vol.17, No.2, pp.445-454, ISSN 0213-3911

Kummar, S.; Fogarasi, M.; Canova, A.; Mota, A. & Ciesielski, T. (2002). Cytokeratin 7 and 20 staining for the diagnosis of lung and colorectal adenocarcinoma. *British Journal of Cancer*, Vol.86, No.12, pp.1884-1887, ISSN 0007-0920

Moll, R.; Franke, W.W. & Schiller, D.L. (1982). The catalog of human cytokeratins: patterns of expression in normal epithelial, tumors and cultured cells. *Cell*, Vol.31, No.1, pp.11-24, ISSN 0092-8674

Moll, R.; Zimbelmann, R.; Goldschmidt, M.D.; Keith, M.; Laufer, J.; Kasper, M.; Koch, P.J. & Franke, W.W. (1993). The human gene encoding cytokeratin 20 and ist expression during fetal development and in gastrointestinal carcinomas. *Differentiation*, Vol.53, No.2, pp.75-93, ISSN 1432-0436

Moll, R.; Divo, M. & Langbein, L. (2008). The human keratins: biology and pathology. *Histochemistry and Cell Biology*, Vol.129, No.6, pp.705-733, ISSN 0948-6143

Nikitakis, N.G.; Tosios, K.I.; Papanikolaou, V.S.; Rivera, H.; Papanicolaou, S.I. & Ioffe, O.B. (2004). Immunohistochemical expression of cytokeratins 7 and 20 in malignant salivary gland tumors. *Modern Pathology*, Vol.17, No.4, pp.407-415, ISSN 0893-3952

Pu, X-Y.; Wang, Z-P.; Chen, Y-R.; Wang, X-H.; Wu, Y-L. & Wang, H-P. (2008). The value of combined use of survivin, cytokeratin 20 and mucin 7 mRNA for bladder cancer detection in voided urine. *Journal of Cancer Research and Clinical Oncology*, Vol.134, No.6, pp.659-665, ISSN 0171-5216

Pujal, J.; Huch, M.; José, A.; Abasolo, I.; Rodolosse, A.; Duch, A.; Sánchez-Palazón, L.; Smith, F.J.D.; McLean, W.H.I.; Fillat, C. & Real, F.X. (2009). Keratin 7 promoter selectively targets transgene expression to normal and neoplastic pancreatic ductal cells *in vitro* and *in vivo*. *The FASEB Journal*, Vol.23, No.5, pp.1366-1375, ISSN 0892-6638

Rekhi, B.; George, S.; Madur, B.; Chinoy, R.F.; Dikshit, R. & Maheshwari, A. (2008). Clinicopathological features and the value of differential cytokeratin 7 and 20 expression in resolving diagnostic dilemmas of ovarian involvement by colorectal adenocarcinoma and vice-versa. *Diagnostic Pathology*, Vol.3, p.39, ISSN 1746-1596

Saeb-Lima, M.; Montante-Montes de Oca, D. & Albores-Saavedra, J. (2008). Merkel cell carcinoma with eccrine differentiation: a clinicopathologic study of 7 cases. *Annals of Diagnostic Pathology*, Vol.12, No.6, pp.410-414, ISSN 1092-9134

Sawan, A.S. (2009). The diagnostic value of immunohistochemistry in the diagnosis of primary and secondary hepatic carcinomas. *The Journal of King Abdulaziz University-Medical Sciences*, Vol.16, No.4, pp.37-48, ISSN 1319-1004

Schweizer, J.; Bowden, P.E.; Coulombe, P.A.; Langbein, L.; Lane, E.B.; Magin, T.M.; Maltais, L.; Omary, M.B.; Parry, D.A.D.; Rogers, M.A. & Wright, M.W. (2006). New consensus nomenclature for mammalian keratins. *The Journal of Cell Biology*, Vol.174, No.2, pp.169-174, ISSN 0021-9525

Simsir, A.; Wei, X-J.; Yee, H.; Moreira, A. & Cangiarella, J. (2004). Differential expression of cytokeratins 7 and 20 and thyroid transcription factor -1 in bronchioloalveolar carcinoma. An immunohistochemical study in fine-needle aspiration biopsy specimens. *American Journal of Clinical Pathology*, Vol.121, No.3, pp.350-357, ISSN 0002-9173

Stopyra, G.A.; Warhol, M.J. & Multhaupt, A.B. (2001). Cytokeratin 20 immunoreactivity in renal oncocytomas. *The Journal of Histochemistry & Cytochemistry*, Vol.49, No.7, pp.919-920, ISSN 0022-1554

Szeverenyi, I.; Cassidy, A.J.; Chung, C.W.; Lee, B.T.; Common, J.E.; Ogg, S.C.; Chen, H.; Sim, S.Y.; Goh, W.L.; Nq, K.W.; Simpson, J.A.; Chee, L.L.; Eng, G.H.; Li, B.; Lunny, D.P.; Chuon, D.; Venkatesh, A.; Khoo, K.H.; McLean, W.H.; Lim, Y.P. & Lane, E.B. (2008). The human intermediate filament database: comprehensive information on a gene family involved in many human diseases. *Human Mutation*, Vol.29, No.3, pp.351-360, ISSN 1059-7794

Tatsumi, N.; Mukaisho, K.; Mitsufuji, S.; Tatsumi, Y.; Sugihara, H.; Okanoue, T. & Hattori, T. (2005). Expression of cytokeratins 7 and 20 in serrated adenoma and related diseases. *Digestive diseases and Sciences*, Vol.50, No.9, pp.1741-1746, ISSN 0163-2116

Tot, T. (2002). Cytokeratins 20 and 7 as biomarkers: usefulness in discriminating primary from metastatic adenocarcinoma. *European Journal of Cancer*, Vol.38, No.6, pp.758-763, ISSN 0959-8049

Upasani, O.S.; Vaidya, M.M. & Bhisey, A.N. (2004). Database on monoclonal antibodies to cytokeratins. *Oral Oncology*, Vol.40, No.3, pp.236-256, ISSN 1368-8375

Wang, J-Y.; Wu, Ch-H.; Lu, Ch-Y.; Hsieh, J-S.; Wu, D-Ch.; Huang, S-Y. & Lin, S-R. (2006). Molecular detection of circulating tumor cells in the peripheral blood of patients with colorectal cancer using RT-PCR: significance of the prediction of postoperative metastasis. *World Journal of Surgery*, Vol.30, No.6, p.1007-1013, ISSN 0364-2313

Wauters, C.C.A.P.; Smedts, F.; Gerrits, L.G.M.; Bosman, F.T. & Ramaekers, F.C.S. (1995). Keratins 7 and 20 as diagnostic markers of carcinomas metastatic to the ovary. *Human Pathology*, Vol.26, No.8, pp.852-855, ISSN 004

5

Cytokeratin 8: The Dominant Type II Intermediate Filament Protein in Lung Cancer

Nobuhiro Kanaji[1,*], Akihito Kubo[2,*], Shuji Bandoh[1], Tomoya Ishii[1], Jiro Fujita[3], Takuya Matsunaga[1] and Etsuro Yamaguchi[2]
[1]Kagawa University
[2]Aichi Medical University School of Medicine
[3]University of the Ryukyus
Japan

1. Introduction

Lung cancer is the leading cause of cancer deaths worldwide. Cytokeratins (CKs) play an important role in cancer biology and circulating forms of CKs have been used as tumor markers in various malignancies. In the present chapter, the biological relevance of CKs and their release into the circulation are discussed, with a focus on CK8, a type II intermediate filament (IF) protein, and its association with type I CKs in lung cancer.

1.1 Lung cancer

Lung cancer is the most common cancer in the world, with an estimated 1.6 million new cases and 1.4 million deaths in 2008. In the United States, 222,000 new lung cancer cases and 157,000 deaths are estimated for 2010 (Jemal et al., 2011). More than four-fifths of all lung cancers are of non-small cell histology, comprised of adenocarcinomas (40-50%), squamous cell carcinomas (25-30%) and large cell carcinomas (10%), while approximately 15% of lung cancers are of small cell histology.

Lung cancer is usually asymptomatic in its early developmental stages, and, even if symptomatic, the symptoms are often non-specific and unrelated to the early stage lung cancer. Accordingly, the majority of lung cancer patients are discovered at inoperable advanced stages. Between 1996 and 2003 in the United States, only 16% of lung cancers were localized when diagnosed (compared with 91% of prostate cancers, 80% of melanomas and 61% of female breast cancers), 35% were locally advanced and 41% were metastatic (Youlden et al., 2008). Most likely because of the aggressive nature of the disease, the prognosis of lung cancer patients remains poor; ranging from a median survival time (MST) of 60 months and a 5-year survival rate of 50% even for the earliest stage IA disease, to an MST of only six months and a 5-year survival rate of as low as 2% in stage IV disease, based on the international database of cases that were classified according to the latest TNM staging system (version 7), which comprised 13,267 cases for clinical stage classification (Goldstraw et al., 2007).

---

* The co-first authors contributed equally to the work

Compared with small cell lung cancer (SCLC), non-small cell lung cancer (NSCLC) is relatively insensitive to cytotoxic chemotherapy and radiotherapy, and surgical resection is highly recommended in the early stages of NSCLC. In locally advanced NSCLC that lies within the radiation field with curative intent, combined modality treatment with chest irradiation and systemic chemotherapy is the standard therapy. If curative thoracic irradiation is not applicable, such as in stage IV disseminated diseases, systemic chemotherapy is the standard care (NCCN.org, 2011).

SCLC is deemed to be a different entity from other lung tumors in terms of its origin, biological behavior, and clinical response to therapeutic interventions. SCLC, which is thought to originate from neuroendocine cells, is a rapidly growing aggressive tumor, and is rarely detected in its early operable stage. The MST of SCLC is mere 2-4 months if no positive treatment is applied (Rodriguez & Lilenbaum, 2010; Simon & Turrisi, 2007). In contrast to its extreme aggressiveness, SCLC is highly sensitive to radiation therapy and chemotherapy. Combination chemo-radiotherapy is the most effective treatment for patients with SCLC of limited extent, whose tumor lies within a radiation field of curative radiotherapy (limited disease, LD), and results in an objective response rate of 80-90% (ORR; % of patients who achieved ≧ 50% tumor volume reduction), an MST of 14-20 months and a 2-year survival rate of 20-40%. However, only palliative chemotherapy is applicable as a positive treatment for patients with disseminated SCLC (extensive disease, ED). ORR, MST and the 2-year survival rate of patients with ED-SCLC are 60-70%, 7-10 months and only less than 5%, respectively(Rodriguez & Lilenbaum, 2010; Simon & Turrisi, 2007).

1.2 Cytokeratins and lung cancer

The cytoskeleton is composed of three different classes of proteins, with different filament diameters: actin microfilaments, tubulin microtubules, and intermediate filaments (IFs) (Quinlan et al., 1985). IF proteins, which are chemically stable filaments of ~10 nm in diameter, constitute cytoskeletal systems in the cytoplasm of most eukaryotic cells. CKs are typical IF proteins that are expressed in a highly epithelial cell-type specific manner. CKs constitute the largest family of proteins, and are subdivided into "acidic" type I (CK9-CK23) and "basic or neutral" type II (CK1-CK8) subclasses (Moll et al., 2008; Moll et al., 1982). These CK subclasses are expressed in epithelial cells in various combinations and form obligate heteropolymers of type I and type II CKs in a tissue- or cell type-specific manner. The dominant IFs expressed in epithelial cells in the respiratory tract are CK8 and CK18, and other type II CKs (5, 6 and 7) as well as type I CKs (17 and 19) are expressed to various extents. CK8 and CK18 expression persists in most carcinomas, whereas other CKs tend to be expressed at lower levels or are lost during tumor progression (Coulombe & Omary, 2002; Oshima, 2002).

The biological functions of CKs, including scaffolding and the maintenance of tissue integrity, have been elucidated through gene knockout studies (Coulombe & Omary, 2002). In addition, CKs play a role in regulating tumorigenesis and tumor invasion in a complex and not yet fully determined manner. Several research groups have reported that co-expression of CK8, CK18 and type III IF vimentin confer highly invasive phenotypes on various tumors (Chu et al., 1993; Chu et al., 1996; Chu et al., 1997; Yamashiro et al., 2010).

However, observations that are apparently contradictory to those mentioned above have also been reported; decreased expression of type I CKs significantly correlated with tumor progression or increased invasion ability in several other tumor types (Buhler & Schaller, 2005; Crowe et al., 1999; Woelfle et al., 2004). The epithelial-mesenchymal transition (EMT) is an embryonic developmental program that is also observed during tumor progression in a variety of cancer types, suggesting that the EMT confers, or potentiates, invasiveness of tumor cells (Takeyama et al., 2010). The roles of CKs in tumor invasion and in the EMT are further discussed later in this chapter.

Although IFs have been assumed to form highly insoluble cytoskeletal networks, CKs are also found in the tumor as well as in the blood, where they have been thought to circulate as a partially degraded complex, which has led to their use as potential tumor markers (Buccheri & Ferrigno, 2001).

Circulating fragments of CK8, CK18 or CK19, such as tissue polypeptide antigen (TPA), tissue polypeptide specific antigen (TPS), Cyfra 21-1, and caspase-cleaved CK18, have been used as tumor markers of various epithelial malignancies (Buccheri & Ferrigno, 2001; Kramer et al., 2004; Pujol et al., 1993). Tumor markers targeting single type I CKs in the systemic circulation have been evaluated: e.g., CK18 as a traditional TPS, caspase-cleaved CK19 as Cyfra 21-1, and the recently developed caspase-cleaved CK18 (M30) as well as total CK18 (M65) (Kramer et al., 2004; Linder et al., 2010). While circulating type II CKs had not been reported as tumor markers targeting single CK origin, we observed that serum levels of a type II CK8 were significantly associated with tumor progression and shortened survival in patients with NSCLC. In the later part of this chapter, we also review the biological relevance and clinical significance of circulating CK-related forms.

2. Expression of cytokeratins in lung cancer

While CKs are expressed in a tissue- or cell-type preferential manner, their expression is also significantly influenced by the differentiation as well as the functional status of cells in a given environment. The expression of IFs in various types of malignant tumors has been extensively evaluated. In most cases, epithelial cancers maintain the characteristic CK expression patterns of the respective tissues and organs from which the cancers were derived. This characteristic enables the use of CKs as diagnostic tools for analysis of tumor pathology (Karantza, 2011; Moll et al., 2008).

2.1 Cytokeratin networks

All eukaryotic cells express actin and tubulin, whereas cytoplasmic IF, the third class of cytoskeletal protein, is only expressed in some metazoans. For example, animals with dermoskeleton usually do not express cytoplasmic IFs. Even in vertebrates, oligodendrocytes, which are a specific type of nerve sheath cell in the central nervous system, do not express such IFs. In cells that do express cytoplasmic IFs, IF proteins have been considered to have an important role in protecting cells from various stresses by adding mechanical strength to the cells.

Nuclear lamins, the so-called type V IF proteins, are believed to be the evolutionary progenitors of the largest family of IF proteins. Lamins are the main structural components of a cage-like structure called the lamina, which is situated underneath the inner nuclear membrane. Although the lamina has quite a different architecture from cytoskeletal networks which are three dimensional and highly branched, the lamina also provides strength to the inner nuclear membrane and supports the shape of the nucleus. Lamin genes are thought to have duplicated several times during metazoan evolution, and these duplicated genes eventually evolved to produce cytoplasmic IFs (Alberts et al., 2008; Hutchison, 2002).

An individual CK subunit is composed of extended CK molecules, each with a central α-helical domain that forms a parallel "coiled-coil" with a CK of the other type (i.e., a type I – type II heterodimer; see also "4. Extracellular Release of Cytokeratins" and Fig. 6). Two CK heterodimers then associate in an antiparallel offset fashion to form a staggered tetramer that associates with another tetramer for further extension of molecules. The tetramer constitutes the soluble CK subunit that is analogous to the actin monomer, or to the αβ-tubulin dimer. The tetramers pack together laterally to form a filament of 10 nm in diameter, which is composed of eight parallel protofilaments assembled from CK tetramers. The large number of polypeptides within the CK filaments has strong lateral hydrophobic interactions that are typical of coiled-coil proteins, which gives CK filaments both elasticity and stability (Alberts et al., 2008).

CK filaments confer mechanical strength to animal cells. Cross-linked keratin networks that are fixed by disulfide bonds exhibit an almost infinite stability, as seen in the outer layer of skin, hair, nails, claws and scales. One single epithelial cell may express multiple types of CKs, and these CKs copolymerize into a single network. CK filaments impart mechanical stability to epithelial tissues in part by anchoring CK filaments at sites of cell-cell contact, called desmosomes, or of cell-matrix contact, called hemidesmosomes (Alberts et al., 2008; Fuchs & Karakesisoglou, 2001).

2.2 Cytokeratin 8 and cytokeratin 18 are the dominant intermediate filament proteins in non-small cell lung cancer

The pair of type II CK8 and type I CK18 is the first CK pair to be detected in early embryonic development. CK8 and CK18 are typically co-expressed and form the primary CK heterodimers in virtually all simple epithelia (one-layered epithelial cells): respiratory epithelia; gastrointestinal epithelia; parenchymatous epithelia including hepatocytes, pancreatic acinar cells, and renal tubular cells; as well as ductal epithelia of parenchymatous organs including bile ducts, renal collecting ducts, and pancreatic ducts. In some types of epithelial cells, e.g., hepatocytes in the liver and acinar cells of the pancreas, the CK8/CK18 pair is the only CK pair expressed. As stated above, CK8 and CK18 are the dominant CK pair in epithelial cells in the respiratory tract, where type II CKs (5, 6 and 7) as well as type I CKs (17 and 19) are also expressed. CK8 and CK18 are CK types that tend to persist in most epithelial cancers (Moll et al., 2008).

Figure 1 shows representative expression patterns of IF proteins in a panel of various cancer cell lines of epithelial and non-epithelial origins, including lung cancer (NSCLC and SCLC), mesothelioma (cancer that develops from the mesothelium, the sac lining the internal body cavities), liver cancer (hepatocellular carcinoma), colorectal cancer, breast cancer, tumors of

T lymphocyte- and B lymphocyte-origins, and a fibroblast-like cell line. We quantified the absolute expression levels of CKs by quantitative immunoblotting (Fig. 1, A and B).

While all NSCLC cell lines express abundant CK8 and CK18 that form the dominant CK pair (~40 pmol per 10^6 cells on average), three out of seven SCLC lines do not express detectable levels of CK8 and CK18, and even when expressed in SCLC, the levels of both CKs were lower than those of NSCLC cells. CK7 and CK19 are usually expressed at lower levels than CK8 and CK18 (respectively ~5 and ~20 pmol per 10^6 cells on average), and are expressed only in a limited number of lung cancer cell lines. None of seven SCLC lines that we screened expressed CK7. Similarly, type I and type II CK messenger RNA (mRNA) expression was previously reported to be higher in NSCLC than SCLC cells (Fukunaga et al., 2002; Ueda et al., 1999). Regarding CK19 expression, two cell lines, HI1017 adenocarcinoma and Lu135 SCLC, do not express CK19 because of a point mutation in the promoter region (at -99, G to C) of the CK19 gene (Fujita et al., 2001). None of the lung cancer cell lines in the panel expressed CK20, which expression was only detected in colorectal cancer cell lines. Other CKs (CK4, CK5, CK6, CK13 and CK17) were not expressed in any lung cancer cell line that we tested (data not shown). These CKs are assumed to be CKs of stratified epithelia (Moll et al., 2008).

NSCLC and SCLC also exhibit differential expression patterns of IF proteins other than type I and type II CKs. Vimentin is a type III IF protein that is expressed in mesenchymal tissues and is presumed to be important for stabilizing the architecture of the cytoplasm. The lymphoid tumors, fibroblast-like cells, and mesothelioma cells tested by immunoblotting all expressed vimentin, as shown in Fig. 1A. The vimentin protein was also detectable by immunoblotting in seven out of 12 NSCLC lines but was not detected in any of the SCLC lines. The absolute expression level of vimentin was 9.8 pmol/10^6 cells on average, approximately one-fourth that of CK8 and CK18. Vimentin was previously reported to be expressed in only ~10% of variant type SCLCs and ~90% of pure SCLCs do not express vimentin (Broers et al., 1986).

Lamins, which are type V IF proteins, are components of the nuclear lamina, an IF network that underlies the inner nuclear membrane and determines the size and shape of the nucleus. Three types of lamins, A, B and C, have been described in mammalian cells (Hutchison, 2002). Lamin A and lamin C, with molecular masses of 74 kDa and 65 kDa respectively, arise from a single gene by alternative splicing (Fisher et al., 1986; McKeon et al., 1986). B-type lamins are represented by lamin B1 and lamin B2 in vertebrates. While A-type lamins are expressed in a developmentally controlled manner, B-type lamins are expressed in all types of cells. Broers examined 22 lung cancer cell lines and 46 fresh frozen lung cancer specimens and reported that B-type lamins were expressed in all of the different cell lines examined, whereas A-type lamins were expressed in all tested NSCLC lines but were absent, or only weakly expressed in 14 out of 16 SCLC cell lines (Broers et al., 1993). Our data confirmed the results of Broers et al.; whereas NSCLCs express lamin A and lamin C at a higher level than SCLCs, lamin B was detected in all cell lines tested. We also noticed that the expression level of lamin B, as determined by quantitative immunoblotting, was significantly higher in SCLC than in NSCLC (mean ± SD, 1.31 ± 0.25 vs. 0.66 ± 0.26, arbitrary units normalized by the intensity of Coomassie staining, $p < 0.05$).

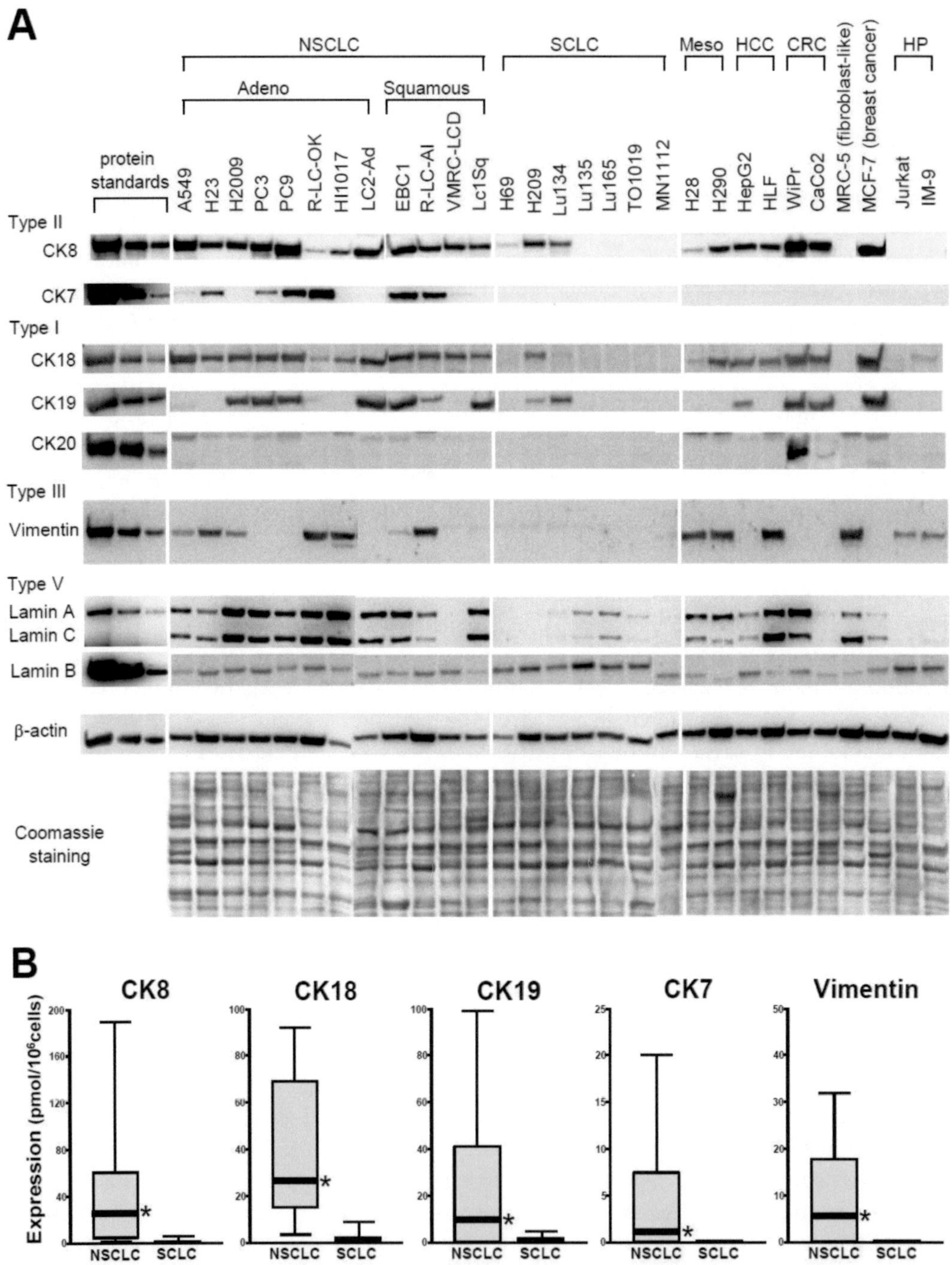

(A) Quantitative immunoblotting of IFs in NSCLC, SCLC and non-lung cancer cell lines.
Of the 19 lung cancer cell lines assayed (12 NSCLC lines; 8 adenocarcinomas, 4 squamous cell carcinomas, and 7 SCLCs), the HI1017, TO1019 and MN1112 lines were established at Kagawa University. The other lung cancer and non-lung cancer cell lines were obtained from the Japan Cancer Research Bank (Tokyo, Japan). The antibodies used were K8.8 (CK8; Neomarkers, Fremont, CA, USA), RCK105 (CK7), Ks18.04

(CK18), Ks19.02 (CK19), Ks20.8 (CK20, all from Progen, Heidelberg, Germany), CIT605 (vimentin, YLEM, Rome, Italy), sc7292 (lamin A/C, Santa-Cruz Biotechnology, Santa Cruz, CA, USA), X223 (nuclear lamin B, Progen), AC-15 (β-actin, Sigma-Aldrich, St Louis, MO, USA), and anti-mouse immunoglobulin G (IgG) conjugated with horseradish peroxidase (HRP; Santa Cruz Biotechnology). Purified protein standards were purchased from Progen. Exponentially growing cells were lysed in 1× sample buffer (62.5 mM Tris-HCl pH 6.8, 2.15% SDS, 5% β-mercaptoethanol, 15% glycerol), and subjected to sodium dodecyl sulfate-polyacrylamide gel electrophoresis (SDS-PAGE) followed by immunoblot analyses using specific antibodies and enhanced chemiluminescence. The PVDF membranes used for immunoblotting were stained with Coomassie Brilliant blue dye to normalize specific signal intensity in immunoblotting. Representative blots of at least three independent experiments are shown.

(B) Absolute expression levels of IF proteins in NSCLC versus SCLC.

The intensity of positive signals in immunoblot analyses was quantified densitometrically using NIH Image version 1.62 (http://rsb.info.nih.gov/nih-image/download.htm). The quantified signal intensities were then compared with those of protein standards at known concentrations. Boxplots indicate median values, ranges of 25-75 percentile and total ranges. *$p < 0.05$ compared with SCLC. Adeno, adenocarcinoma; Squamous, squamous cell carcinoma; Meso, mesothelioma; HCC, hepatocellular carcinoma; CRC, colorectal carcinoma; HP, hematopoietic tumors.

Fig. 1. Expression of IFs in non-small cell lung cancer (NSCLC), small cell lung cancer (SCLC) and non-lung cancer.

2.3 Mechanisms for maintaining cytokeratin filament networks

Compared with the intensively studied actin filaments or microtubules, the mechanism of assembly and disassembly of IFs is not well understood. However, several types of IFs exhibit a highly dynamic structure in metazoan cells. Type III vimentin is probably the most intensively studied cytoplasmic IF. Similar to the mechanism by which phosphorylation regulates the disassembly of nuclear lamins, vimentin structures also disassemble during the mitosis phase of the cell division cycle following specific phosphorylation of vimentin at its amino-terminus by cyclin-dependent kinase 1 (Chou et al., 1990; Sihag et al., 2007). Phosphorylation is also considered to alter the solubility of IF proteins including both types of CKs (Ku et al., 2002; Liao & Omary, 1996). One of the IF-interacting proteins, 14-3-3 is involved in CK solubilization during mitosis by binding to the phosphorylated serine residue (Ser 33) of CK18 (Ku et al., 2002).

A single epithelial cell often express more than two types of CKs, and all of these CKs copolymerize into a single CK network. One good example of such copolymerization is seen in lung cancer NSCLC cells. Since NSCLC cells originate from the respiratory tract, they express CK8 and CK18 as their primary CK pair and also frequently express CK7 and CK19 as their secondary CKs (Fig. 1, A). These observations raise the question as to why one cell expresses multiple type I and type II CKs. One can easily hypothesize that multiple CKs would compensate for each other if expression of a particular CK was disrupted. We show the results of simple experiments to test this hypothesis (Fig. 2. Modified with permission from (Kanaji et al., 2007)).

A549 cells express CK8 and CK18 as the dominant CK pair and also express CK7 at a lower level and CK19 at a minute, trace level. Roughly equimolar amounts of type I and type II CKs are expressed in these cells (Fig. 2, A), which is consistent with previous observations (Kim et al., 1984). In this simplistic model, we regarded CKs as being in a filament form (i.e., insoluble), although a small fraction (~5%) of the total CK has been reported to be soluble (Chou et al., 1993). This model implies that the dominant type I/type II CK pair (depicted as large discs) likely plays a central role in the formation of CK networks. For example, CK8/CK18 seems to be the most important pair in A549 cells, whereas CK8/CK19, CK7/CK18, and CK7/CK19 are present as minor pairs. Based on these observations we also hypothesized that maintenance of the dominant CK pair is critical for the integrity of CK networks. Thus, a decrease in a dominant CK of one type, may also lead to decreases in CKs of the complementary type because of filament instability. Furthermore, if levels of a dominant CK decrease, another CK of the same type would increase to prevent disruption of the CK network. To test these hypotheses, RNA interference was used to knockdown expression of CK genes in this cell line.

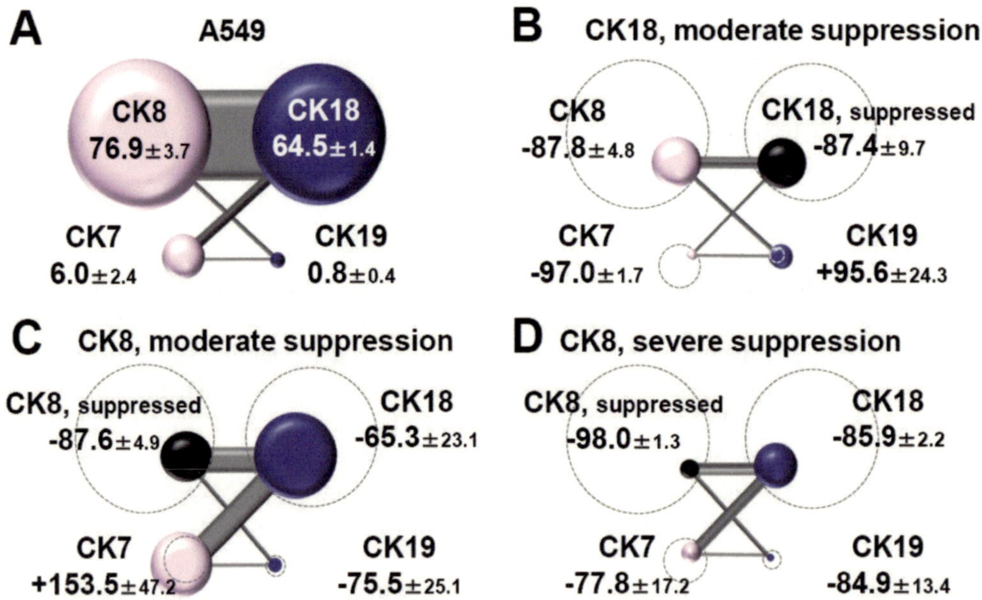

(A) Schematic outline of the experiment. The expression levels of CK proteins in the NSCLC A549 cell line were evaluated by quantitative immunoblotting. CK protein levels are shown as means ± S.D. (pmol/10^6 cells) of three independent experiments. The thickness of the lines connecting type I and type II CKs represents their putative binding capacities based on the calculated molar ratios of CKs of each CK type. (B-D) CK levels and putative binding were similarly measured after CK gene suppression by RNA interference. CK protein levels following RNA interference were quantified and are shown compared with those of parent cells (transfection with control short interfering RNA; dotted circle). The black discs represent expression levels of CKs targeted by specific RNA interference. Numbers are % changes of expression levels from those of control cells (mean ± S.D.).

Fig. 2. Quantitative evaluation of type I and type II CKs upon single CK suppression

When expression of the type I CK18 was knocked-down to a moderate degree (Fig. 2, B), protein expression of both of the type II CKs, CK8 and CK7, was also considerably suppressed. In contrast, a slight but clear increment in protein expression of the other type I CK, CK19, was detected, suggesting compensatory up-regulation of the non-targeted CK19. We confirmed that only the mRNA expression of CK18, and not that of other CKs, was severely diminished following RNA interference targeting of CK18, indicating that the changes in the protein expression of CK8, CK7 and CK19 were changes at the protein level and were not due to off-target effects of the short interfering RNA (siRNA) that targeted CK18. Similarly, when type II CK8 was suppressed to a moderate degree (Fig. 2, C), protein expression of both of the type I CKs, CK18 and CK19, was decreased but, conversely, the type II CK7 was up-regulated, at the protein level, thereby decreasing the damage on total type II CKs. However, this compensatory mechanism that maintained total CK integrity was almost completely disrupted when expression of the dominant CK8 was severely suppressed (Fig. 2, D).

Therefore, to maintain properly functioning CK networks, there appears to be a requirement for a certain "threshold" level of expression of a single dominant CK. If the expression level of the dominant CK is lower than this threshold, then type I-II pairing, and, accordingly, elongation of IF protofibrils or filaments, cannot occur and CK networks cannot be formed. Redundant expression of multiple CKs seems to be advantageous for the stabilization of CK networks, and the above observations may explain, at least in part, why a single cell expresses multiple type I and type II CKs (Kanaji et al., 2007).

3. Cytokeratins in tumor invasiveness and epithelial-mesenchymal transition

3.1 Relationship between cytokeratin expression levels and cancer invasiveness

Several functions of CKs, including roles in scaffolding and tissue integrity, have been demonstrated in normal tissues using gene knockout studies (Coulombe & Omary, 2002; Karantza, 2011; Moll et al., 2008). In addition, it has been reported that CKs play a role in the regulation of cancer cell invasion, metastasis and tumorigenesis (Buhler & Schaller, 2005; Chu et al., 1993; Chu et al., 1996; Chu et al., 1997; Crowe et al., 1999; Hendrix et al., 1992; Kanaji et al., 2011; Schaller et al., 1996; Woelfle et al., 2004; Yamashiro et al., 2010). Table 1 summarizes published studies that describe the correlation of endogenous CK expression with cancer invasiveness.

Author, year	Cancer type	Endogenous CKs expressed	Invasive or metastatic phenotype
Hendrix, 1992	Melanoma (cell lines)	CK8 and 18	High
Schaller, 1996	Breast cancer (clinical tumors and cell lines)	CK18	Low
Chu, 1997	Lung adenocarcinoma (cell line)	CK8 and 18	High
Crowe, 1999	Oral squamous cell carcinoma (cell line)	CK19	Low
Woelfle, 2004	Breast cancer (patients)	CK18	Longer survival
Yamashiro, 2010	Cutaneous squamous cell carcinoma (patients)	CK8 and 18	High
Kanaji, 2011	Lung adenocarcinoma (cell lines)	CK7, 8, 18 and 19	Low

Table 1. Correlation of endogenous CK expression with cancer invasiveness

In 1992, expression levels of CK8 and CK18 were determined in nine human melanoma cell lines expressing vimentin. The expression of CK8 and CK18 was below the level of detection in the poorly metastatic A375P cell line, was at a low level in the moderately metastatic A375M line, and displayed the highest level in the highly metastatic C8161 line (Hendrix et al., 1992). Subpopulations of the human lung adenocarcinoma cell line CL1 were selected according to their invasive ability that was assessed using a Transwell invasion chamber assay. These subpopulations showed a 4- to 6-fold increase in their ability to invade a basement membrane matrix over that of their parental cells and expressed higher levels of the 92 kDa gelatinase, vimentin, CK8 and CK18. In addition, clonal isolation of anti-CK18-antibody-positive and -negative cell populations demonstrated that expression of CK18 correlated with their enhanced invasive ability (Chu et al., 1997). CK8 and 18 are not expressed in normal keratinocytes. However, both CKs are co-expressed in a metastatic derivative of a transformed mouse keratinocyte cell line in which they formed CK8/18 filaments (Yamashiro et al., 2010). In addition, analysis of specimens from 21 pre-invasive and 24 invasive cutaneous squamous cell carcinomas (cSCCs) derived from patients indicated that ectopic CK8/18 coexpression was almost exclusively detected in invasive cSCCs (Yamashiro et al., 2010).

In contrast, several reports have shown an inverse correlation between CK expression levels and cancer invasiveness or progression. Oral squamous cell carcinoma (SCC) lines that did not express CK19 were significantly more invasive *in vitro* than those which retained CK19 expression (Crowe et al., 1999). CK18 protein expression was low in highly metastatic breast cancer cell lines, but, conversely, was high in weakly metastatic cell lines (Schaller et al., 1996). We have recently established invasive sublines of NSCLC adenocarcinoma cells, HI1017 and A549, by repeated selection of invasive cells using Matrigel, a membrane invasion chamber system (Kanaji et al., 2011). In this *in vitro* invasion assay, invasive sublines of these cells showed very much higher invasive ability compared with that of the parental HI1017 and A549 cells (>100-fold and ~50-fold, respectively, $p < 0.01$) as shown in Fig. 3 (Figures 3–5. Modified with permission from (Kanaji et al., 2011)). These invasive sublines showed lower CK expression levels than their parental cells.

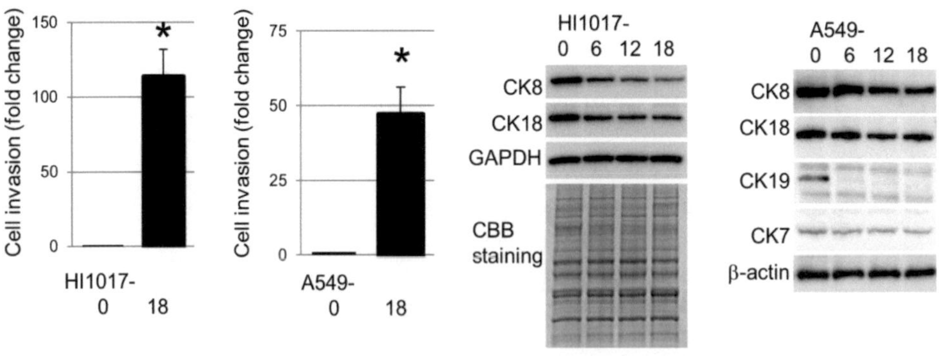

Highly invasive sublines of the NSCLC cell lines, HI1017 and A549, designated as HI1017-18 and A549-18 respectively, were selected by repeated assay (up to 18 times) of cell invasion, which was assessed using an *in vitro* invasion assay with Matrigel-coated membranes. CK expression was determined by quantitative immunoblotting as described in Fig. 1. Repeated MICS-selection of HI1017 and A549 cells resulted in decreased CK expression levels. HI1017-18 and A549-18 show lower CK expression levels than their respective parental cells (HI1017-0 and A549-0). *$p < 0.01$ compared with HI1017-0 or A549-0.

Fig. 3. Increased invasive ability and decreased CK expression of cells selected using a Matrigel membrane invasion chamber system (MICS).

The correlation between CK expression and survival has also been examined. CK18 protein expression was immunohistochemically examined using paraffin sections of primary breast carcinoma tumors from 134 patients. The mortality rate was 4.5% in the CK18 immunostaining-positive group and 44.6% in the CK18-negative group during an 8-year follow up period. CK18 expression was an independent and significant predictor for overall survival by a multivariate analysis (Schaller et al., 1996). Woelfle et al. evaluated the expression pattern of CK18 in 1,458 primary breast cancers by immunohistochemical analysis using a high-density tissue microarray. CK18 expression was similarly downregulated in 25.4% of human breast cancers compared to normal breast tissues. Down-regulation of CK18 significantly correlated with advanced tumor stages and pathologically higher grades. Kaplan-Meier survival analysis revealed that CK18 expression was a prognostic indicator of both overall survival (p=0.015) and cancer-specific survival (p=0.005). Based on the correlation between tumor CK18 expression and patient prognosis the authors concluded that low CK18 expression may be an indicator of poor prognosis and that CK18 might suppress tumor progression (Schaller et al., 1996).

3.2 Altered expression levels of cytokeratins and cancer invasiveness

Table 2 summarizes published studies that analyzed the effect of CK inhibition or overexpression on invasive or metastatic phenotypes of cancer cell lines

Author, year	Cancer type	Manipulation of CK expression	Change in invasive or metastatic potential
Hendrix, 1992	Melanoma	Inhibition of CK18	Decreased
Chu, 1993	Mouse fibroblast	Induction of CK8 and 18	Increased
Chu, 1996	Melanoma	Induction of CK8 and 18	Increased
Crowe, 1999	Oral squamous cell carcinoma	Induction of CK19	Decreased
Bühler, 2005	Breast cancer	Induction of CK18	Decreased
Kanaji, 2011	Lung adenocarcinoma	Induction of CK19	Decreased
		Inhibition of CK8 and 18	Increased

Table 2. Effect of modification of CK expression on cancer invasiveness

Disruption of CK in human melanoma cells by transfection with a mutant CK18 complementary DNA (cDNA) resulted in decreased invasive and metastatic potential that directly correlated with a reduction in migratory activity (Hendrix et al., 1992). Mouse L cells, which are fibroblasts that express vimentin, were transfected with both CK8 and 18. Cells that expressed exogenous CK8/18 filaments showed a higher migratory activity on, and higher ability to invade, extracellular matrix-coated filters compared with the parental and control-transfected clones. Furthermore, a heterogeneous population of L clones that were selected using serial migration assays were enriched in CK-positive cells (Chu et al., 1993). An A375P human melanoma cell line that expressed vimentin and had low invasive ability was transfected with CK8 and CK18 cDNA. The resultant stable transfectants that expressed vimentin and the two CKs, showed a two to three-fold increase in their invasion of basement membrane matrix and migration through gelatin *in vitro* compared to non-transfected cells (Chu et al., 1996). Similarly, Yamashiro et al also reported that coexpression of exogenous CK8 and CK18 conferred invasiveness to the parental non-metastatic transformed mouse keratinocyte line (Yamashiro et al., 2010).

In contrast, there have been several reports that overexpression of CKs can reduce cancer invasiveness. Stable expression of CK19 cDNA in CK19 negative SCC cell lines of the head and neck altered cell morphology and intercellular adhesiveness, and significantly decreased the number of cells able to migrate through a reconstituted basement membrane (Crowe et al., 1999). A dramatic reduction in the aggressiveness of the breast cancer cell line MDA-MB-231 was observed following forced CK18 expression (Buhler & Schaller, 2005). We transfected exogenous CK19 cDNA into the lung adenocarcinoma cell line HI1017 that lacks endogenous CK19 (Kanaji et al., 2011). The resulting CK19-expressing clones showed lower invasive ability than mock-transfected cells (Fig. 4).

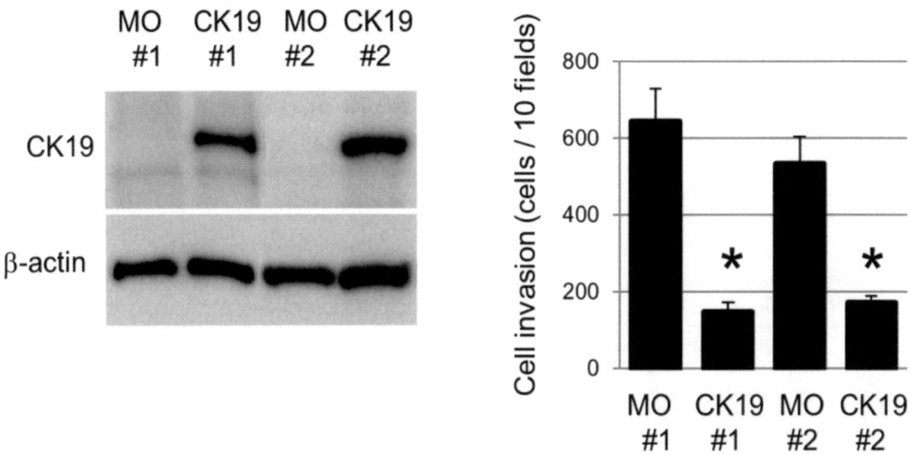

(Left) Western blotting of CK19 expression in stable HI1017 clones #1 and #2 expressing exogenous CK19. (Right) Invasion assay. Data are means ± S.D. of three independent experiments. *$p < 0.01$ compared with mock (MO) transfections.

Fig. 4. Exogenous CK19 inhibits the invasive phenotype.

In addition, suppression of either CK8 or CK18 by short interfering RNAs led to a decrease in total CKs and increased invasiveness of both of HI1017 and A549 cell lines (Fig. 5, (Kanaji et al., 2011)).

These apparently contradictory observations regarding CK expression and tumor progression might suggest that CKs may function differently depending on the tissue and the cellular context. Another important IF protein which may affect invasive ability is vimentin. Invasive lung cancer cell lines strongly expressed vimentin as well as CKs (Chu et al., 1997). Interestingly, forced CK18 expression was associated with a complete loss of vimentin in a breast cancer cell line and resulted in a reduced malignant potential (Buhler & Schaller, 2005). Therefore, in addition to the expression level of CKs, the negative correlation of CKs and vimentin could also play an important role in cancer invasion.

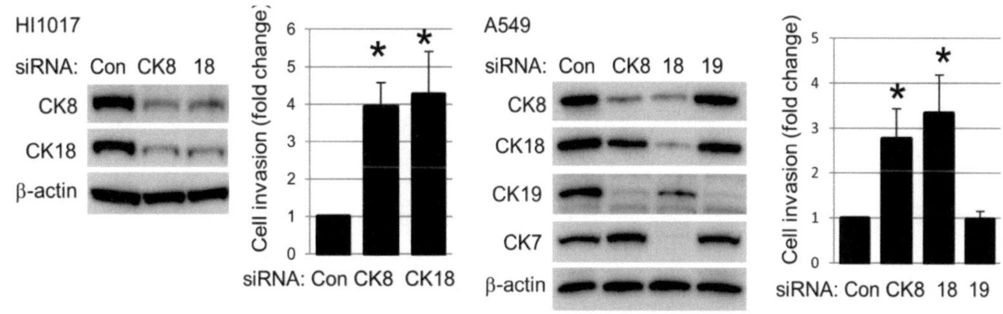

HI1017 and A549 cell lines were transfected with siRNA targeting CK8, CK18 or CK19 and were subjected to an invasion assay and to immunoblotting to confirm silencing efficacy. $^*p < 0.05$ compared with control siRNA (Con).

Fig. 5. Inhibition of CK8 and 18 results in a decrease in invasive ability of lung cancer cell lines.

3.3 Epithelial-mesenchymal transition (EMT) and cytokeratins

A developmental regulatory program, referred to as the "epithelial-mesenchymal transition" (EMT), has been strongly suggested to be a mechanism by which transformed epithelial cells can acquire the ability to invade, to resist apoptosis and to disseminate. Indeed EMT traits have been reported to be involved in embryonic development and to confer invasiveness to cancer cells during the progression of cancer (Hanahan & Weinberg, 2011; Takeyama et al., 2010). Various types of factors have been reported to induce EMT, including cytokines, growth factors and anti-cancer drugs (Kasai et al., 2005; Li et al., 2009; Shih & Yang, 2011; Yee et al., 2010). In A549 lung adenocarcinoma cells, which retain the properties of type II lung alveolar epithelial cells, EMT was induced by transforming growth factor-β1 (TGF-β1), and this induction was accompanied by morphological change into a spindle fibroblast-like shape, an increase in mesenchymal markers including vimentin, fibronectin, collagens I and III, and connective tissue growth factor (CTGF), and a decrease in epithelial markers including E-cadherin and CK19 (Kasai et al., 2005). Doxorubicin could induce EMT in cells of the breast cancer cell line MCF7, which also retain several characteristics of differentiated mammary epithelium, as evidenced by doxorubicin-mediated increases in alpha-smooth muscle actin (α-SMA) and vimentin and decreases in E-cadherin and CK19 (Li et al., 2009). Similarly, down-regulation of the epithelial markers E-cadherin and CK8 and 18 was observed in EMT-induced prostate cancer cells (Yee et al., 2010). In addition to the down-regulation of several epithelial markers of differentiation such as E-cadherin, CKs were also down-regulated during the EMT process in these types of tumors.

Down-regulation of CKs may also be related to EMT in clinical colorectal tumors. Knosel et al have recently reported that a low CK expression level correlates with a shortened survival time. Using tissue microarrays comprised of 468 colorectal cancers from 203 patients, and an unsupervised hierarchical clustering analysis, they discovered subgroups of colorectal cancers that were characterized by reduced CK8 and 20 expression, and that differed from the other groups by a shorter patient survival time. Evaluation of specific biomarkers by Kaplan-Meier analysis showed that reduced CK8 expression ($p < 0.01$) was significantly associated with a shorter patient survival time. They concluded that reduced coexpression of CK8 and CK20 may indicate the occurrence of an EMT in the development of more aggressive colorectal cancers (Knosel et al., 2006).

Cell migration is necessary for cancer invasion into the surrounding stroma. Another factor important for invasion is degradation of the extracellular matrix by matrix metalloproteases (MMPs). During EMT, the expression of junction proteins is lost along with other epithelial characteristics, which results in a loss of the ability of tumor cells to interact with each other, thereby promoting a migratory phenotype (Fuxe et al., 2010). Indeed, loss of desmosomal proteins has been shown to increase epithelial cell migration (Rieger-Christ et al., 2005; South et al., 2003). CKs connect with desmosomes to form extensive cadherin-mediated cytoskeletal structures (Buhler & Schaller, 2005; Kouklis et al., 1994; Smith & Fuchs, 1998). These data would therefore be consistent with the idea that the loss of CK expression can promote an invasive phenotype through a mechanism that elevates migratory ability by down-regulating desmosomal proteins. In agreement with this hypothesis, it was reported that transfection of CK19 into squamous cell carcinoma cells led to a decrease in invasiveness due to a reduced migratory ability (Crowe et al., 1999). In addition, CK18-transfected breast cancer cells showed low invasive ability because the expressed exogenous CK18 dimerized with endogenous CK8, and resulted in the up-regulation of two desmosomal proteins, desmoglein and plakoglobin as well as E-cadherin (Buhler & Schaller, 2005).

In parallel with the above-described effects, cells undergoing EMT boost their migratory capacity through increased expression of mesenchymal proteins including vimentin and α-SMA (Fuxe et al., 2010). Overexpression of vimentin in cancer correlates well with accelerated tumor growth, invasion, and poor prognosis (Satelli & Li, 2011). Interestingly, a decrease in vimentin expression was observed in breast cancer cells transfected with CK18 (Buhler & Schaller, 2005). There may be mutually exclusive expression of CKs and vimentin in situations such as EMT, and up-regulation of vimentin could be one possible mechanism by which loss of CKs induces the migratory and invasive ability of cancer cells.

Thus, tumor cells undergoing EMT acquire the capacity to migrate and invade the surrounding stroma and subsequently spread via blood and lymphatic vessels to distant sites (Fuxe et al., 2010). Accumulating evidence will further enhance our understanding of an important role of CKs in EMT-induced cancer progression.

4. Extracellular release of cytokeratins

Until recently even a large number of biomedical researchers found it difficult to believe that highly stable cytoskeletal proteins are released from the cytoplasm into the extracellular space. However, the organization of the IF network is extremely dynamic and IF proteins are indeed released extracellularly through several mechanisms. Post-translational modifications of CKs, the presence of soluble CK pools, and disruption as well as reorganization of cell membranes and/or CK networks, all appear to contribute to the extracellular release of highly insoluble CKs (Coulombe & Omary, 2002; Karantza, 2011; Omary et al., 2006).

4.1 Post-translational modification of cytokeratins and the soluble cytokeratin pool

The type I and type II CKs, as well as other cytoplasmic IF proteins, consist of a common tripartite domain structure, with non-helical amino terminal (head) and carboxyl terminal (tail) domains that flank a central α-helical rod domain consisting of~310 amino acids. The amino acid sequence of the rod domain is highly conserved, whereas the size and sequence of the amino-terminal head and carboxyl-terminal tail domains vary extensively between individual IFs. Type I and type II CKs associate to form obligate heterodimers, and anti-parallel heterodimers (referred to as tetramers) polymerize in a staggered fashion to form protofilaments (3 nm in diameter), which unite to form protofibrils (4- 5 nm in diameter), and then to IFs (10 nm in diameter) (Fig. 6; also see "2.1 Cytokeratin networks"). This IF structure that is 10 nm in diameter exhibits remarkable chemical stability, resisting high temperature, high salt and detergent solubilization (Alberts et al., 2008; Steinert et al., 1993).

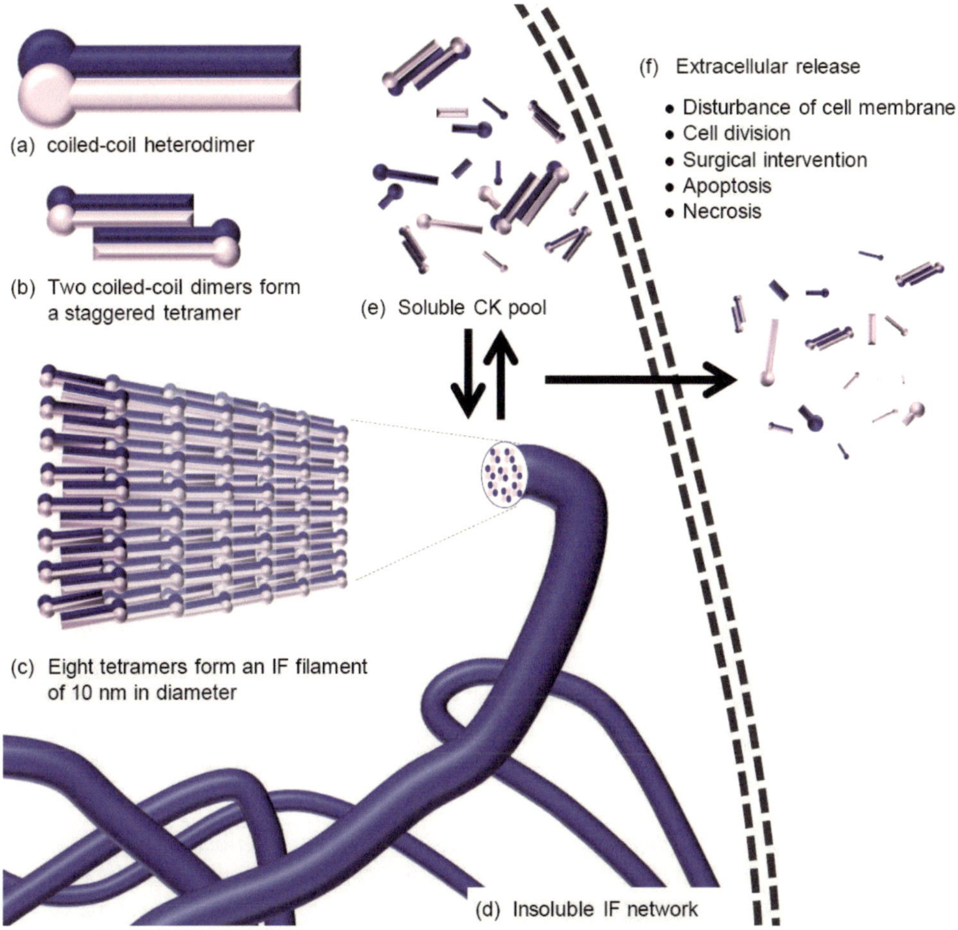

(a) Two different types (type I and type II) of CK monomers (the COOH-terminals are drawn as balls for orientation) pair in parallel through the central rod domain, termed the α-helical region, of each monomer, forming a "coiled-coil heterodimer."
(b) Two dimers form an antiparallel tetramer of four polypeptide chains. This tetramer is the fundamental soluble subunit of cytokeratin IFs. Within each tetramer, the two dimers are mutually offset allowing one tetramer to associate with another tetramer.
(c) Tetramers line up together, with eight tetramers in a cross section, ultimately forming a filament that is 10-nm in diameter, which is the component polypeptide of the insoluble IF network (d)
(e) A small fraction of total CKs form a soluble pool in the cytoplasm.
(f) Upon cell division, cell death (apoptosis or necrosis) or disruption of the cell membrane, the soluble fraction of CKs is released into the circulation.

Fig. 6. Extracellular release of IF proteins

IF proteins, such as type III vimentin and type IV neurofilaments, undergo phosphorylation during the G2/M phase of the cell cycle, which plays a key role in the assembly and disassembly of IF subunits (Sihag et al., 2007). Both type I and type II CKs also undergo phosphorylation. Chou et al. first reported that asynchronously growing human colon cancer HT29 cells (G0/G1 phase of the cell cycle) have a substantial pool of soluble CK that constitutes ~5% of the total cellular CK. Several other cell lines showed a similar, significant pool of soluble cytosolic CK8/CK18. The arrest of cells in the G2/M phase of the cell cycle was associated with a concurrent increase in CK solubility. CK8/CK18 was shown to be in dimeric or tetrameric forms, but primarily in tetrameric keeping the ability of assembly (Chou et al., 1993; Omary et al., 2006). Subsequently, Liao et al. demonstrated that CK-associated 14-3-3 proteins act as a soluble co-factor by binding to phosphorylated CK8/CK18 and sequestering them into a soluble fraction. In case of vimentin, the phosphorylation-induced disassembly of vimentin filaments results in the release of tetrameric subunits, suggesting that assembly and disassembly are phosphorylation-regulated events (Eriksson et al., 2004). Thus, the majority of CK8 and CK18 molecules form an insoluble CK network during the G1 phase of the cell cycle. During the S phase and the G2/M phase, CK8 and CK18 become hyperphosphorylated, resulting in an increase in the soluble pool of CKs. Dephosphorylation of CKs at the end of mitosis returns CK8 and CK18 into a G1 cytoskeletal network (Liao & Omary, 1996; Omary et al., 2006).

4.2 Mechanisms of cytokeratin release

Several mechanisms by which insoluble macromolecule IF network components are released into the circulation, have been suggested. In these mechanisms the presence of soluble CK pools, as well as disruption and reorganization of cell membranes and/or CK networks appear to contribute to the extracellular release of largely insoluble CKs (Chou et al., 1993; Omary et al., 2006). CKs have been found in extracellular spaces both *in vitro* and *in vivo*, in conditioned culture medium to circulating human blood. CK release is observed during cell growth/cell divisions, after surgical intervention, and upon cell death induction (e.g., radiation therapy and/or cytotoxic chemotherapy) (Bauer et al., 1986; Bjorklund & Bjorklund, 1983; Brabon et al., 1984; Caulin et al., 1997; Dohmoto et al., 2000; Dohmoto et al., 2001; Sheard et al., 2002; Tinnemans et al., 1995).

CKs are released during cell division. In early 1980s, Bjorklund reported that in cultured uterine cervix cancer HeLa cells, TPA (i.e. CK8, CK18 and CK19) is seen in perinuclear area during the early S phase. After cell division TPA becomes externalized leaving the cell free of visible TPA, while TPA levels in the culture medium increase at this stage (Bjorklund & Bjorklund, 1983). Upon estrogen stimulation, breast cancer MCF-7 cells release CKs, part of which localized to the cell surface, into the tissue culture medium (Brabon et al., 1984). TPA is found in the systemic circulation during perioperative period. Twenty patients with lung cancer or gastric cancer who underwent curative surgery were prospectively monitored for serum TPA prior to surgery and during the subsequent year. Serum levels of TPA immediately fell after surgery, and following the initial 2 weeks after complete removal of tumors, serum TPA rise to some extent. This temporal increment is interpreted as being caused by tissue repair and cell proliferation (Bauer et al., 1986).

Post-translational modification and protein processing on CKs during apoptosis have been intensively studied. CK aggregation in the cytoplasm is one of earliest events of apoptosis in epithelial cells, while at a later stage CKs degrade (Tinnemans et al., 1995). These CK filament reorganizations during apoptosis are accompanied by caspase cleavage of type I CKs (Caulin et al., 1997). Using MCF-7 cells, Sheard et al. revealed TPS (i.e., CK18) and Cyfra 21-1 (CK19) are abundantly released during apoptosis and the release precedes DNA fragmentation (Sheard et al., 2002). We also observed mRNA expression of CK19 is essential in Cyfra 21-1 formation and caspase 3 plays an important role in producing Cyfra 21-1 in human lung cancer cell lines (Dohmoto et al., 2000; Dohmoto et al., 2001). Kramer described that large amounts of CK18 are released into extracellular space during necrosis induced by oligomycin, and that release of CK18 is a marker of epithelial cell death and not a marker of apoptosis (Kramer et al., 2004).

5. Circulating cytokeratins and their clinical significance

Clinically, circulating molecules related to CK8, CK18 or CK19 have widely been used as tumor markers of various types of malignancies. Here we briefly review CK-related tumor markers and discuss issues to be considered when evaluating circulating CK-related molecules, focusing especially on CK8.

5.1 Circulating cytokeratin-related molecules and their biological and clinical relevance

CK-related circulating polypeptides have served as useful tumor markers of various epithelial malignancies. Measurement of CKs in the circulation is clinically useful for the early detection of recurrence, and for assessment of the disease response to treatment. The most widely applied CK tests are the monoclonal antibody-based assays: TPA, TPS and Cyfra 21-1.

TPA has long been used as a serological marker in various types of epithelial malignancies, e.g., lung cancer, breast cancer, colorectal cancer, head and neck cancer, and urothelial cancer (Bennink et al., 1999; Gion et al., 2000; Nicolini et al., 1995; Plebani et al., 1995; Rosati et al., 2000; Soletormos et al., 2004). TPA is a good example of a broad-spectrum CK assay, and measures CK8, CK18 and CK19 in serum samples. TPA was reported to be a highly sensitive marker of cancer patients (Mellerick et al., 1990). However, in contrast, Anquilina reported that although TPA has both a sensitivity and a specificity of 65%, this may not be sufficient for discrimination between malignant and benign lung diseases (Aquilina et al., 1992).

TPS assay was proposed as an advance over TPA assay. It was claimed that serum TPS levels correlated highly with the proliferation rate of cancer cells (Buccheri & Ferrigno, 2001). Studies of patients with lung diseases of either neoplastic or non-neoplastic origin revealed TPS sensitivity rates between 13–54% (Correale et al., 1994; Giovanella et al., 1995; Nisman et al., 1998; Pujol et al., 1994; Pujol et al., 1996; van der Gaast et al., 1994). TPS sensitivity did not vary in NSCLC with different histology, but it did differ according to the progression of lung cancer (Giovanella et al., 1995; Pujol et al., 1996).

Cyfra 21-1 is an assay that uses two monoclonal antibodies to measure soluble CK19 fragments in the circulation, (Pujol et al., 1993). Cyfra 21-1 has been most intensively studied in lung cancer and head and neck cancer (Nisman et al., 1998; Yen et al., 1998). Our hypothesis regarding the mechanism of Cyfra 21-1 production was that Cyfra 21-1 release depends on CK19 expression and cell apoptosis. We tested this hypothesis using 13 lung cancer cell lines. The mRNA expression level of CK19 in these cells significantly correlated with the levels of Cyfra 21-1 in culture supernatants as measured by ELISA, as well as with intracellular protein expression of CK19 assessed by immunoblotting, and with immunopositivity of CK19 in immunohistochemical analysis. Furthermore, a specific inhibitor of caspase 3 efficiently inhibited the release of Cyfra 21-1 into culture supernatants. Based on these observations we concluded that caspase 3 plays an important role in the production of Cyfra 21-1 in lung cancer cell lines (Dohmoto et al., 2001). Pujol et al evaluated Cyfra 21-1 and TPS in 405 lung cancer patients (91 SCLC and 314 NSCLC) and in 59 patients with non-malignant lung diseases. Receiver operating characteristics (ROC) analysis, in which both the sensitivity and specificity of Cyfra 21-1 and TPS were continually examined, demonstrated that Cyfra 21-1 assay was more accurate than TPS assay for detection of both SCLC and NSCLC. The sensitivity of Cyfra 21-1 was highest for squamous cell carcinoma (0.61) and lowest for SCLC (0.36), whereas the sensitivity of TPS did not vary among histological types (overall sensitivity, 0.40). The values of both Cyfra 21-1 and TPS significantly reflected the disease stage in NSCLC. However, when multivariate analysis was performed to take into account other significant factors, only Cyfra 21-1, and not TPS, was confirmed to be an independent prognostic factor (Pujol et al., 1996).

CK18 is a useful tumor marker as evidenced by TPA and TPS assays. Type I CK18 is also a good substrate for caspases as discussed earlier in this chapter. ELISAs are now available for assay of CK18 that is cleaved at Asp396 by caspases, which can be detected using M30 and M5 monoclonal antibodies (referred to as M30), and for assay of total CK18, which can be detected using M5 and M6 monoclonal antibodies (referred to as M65) (Kramer et al., 2004; Linder et al., 2010). M30-recognized circulating CK18 is released from apoptotic cells, whereas M65-recognized CK18 reflects cell death by any cause. The ratio of caspase-cleaved to total CK18, calculated using M30- and M65-ELISAs, may provide potentially useful information regarding the mode of tumor cell death (Linder et al., 2010). The usefulness of M30 for tumor monitoring has been demonstrated by Koelink et al. They determined caspase-cleaved CK18 and total CK18 levels in the plasma of 49 colorectal cancer patients, before and after surgical resection. Both the levels of caspase-cleaved CK18 and total CK18 were related to disease stage and tumor diameter. The M30/M65 ratio decreased with tumor progression, and was also predictive of disease free survival (Koelink et al., 2009). De Petris et al. measured circulating total CK18, caspase-cleaved CK18 and Cyfra 21-1 in 200 healthy blood donors, 113 patients with non-malignant lung diseases and 179 NSCLC cases, using ELISA assays. The diagnostic accuracy of both CK18 forms in distinguishing between NSCLC and healthy blood donors was 56%, whereas it was 94% for Cyfra 21-1. Multivariate survival analysis revealed that total CK18 was a better prognostic factor than Cyfra 21-1 or caspase-cleaved CK18. The reason why caspase-cleaved CK18 was not of prognostic value might be due, at least in part, to the greater importance of tumor necrosis compared to tumor apoptosis in this disease (De Petris et al., 2011).

The above single measurements of circulating type I CKs have significant value for the diagnosis and monitoring of patients with NSCLC. However, a single measurement of circulating type II CKs has not been reported as tumor markers, which prompted us to determine the clinical significance of circulating CK8 in NSCLC.

5.2 Cytokeratin 8 as a novel tumor marker

As described above, type II CK8 is the dominant CK in NSCLC, and circulating CK-related species have been used as a valuable tumor marker in the clinic. We hypothesized that the levels of circulating CK8 would be higher in patients with NSCLC than in patients with SCLC, and that circulating CK8 would be related to disease progression, metastases, and survival in patients with NSCLC. To test this hypothesis, we determined the serum levels of CK8 in patients with lung cancer (Fukunaga et al., 2002).

We first established an ELISA assay of CK8 using the anti-CK8 monoclonal antibody M20. We next determined the CK8 mRNA expression level of 9 NSCLC cell lines (7 adenocarcinomas and 2 squamous cell carcinomas) and 9 SCLC cell lines using a semi-quantitative competitive reverse transcription-polymerase chain reaction (RT-PCR). The expression levels of CK8 mRNA were significantly higher in NSCLC cells compared with those in SCLC cells (mean ± standard error: 60.8 ± 16.2 versus 9.9 ± 2.5 attomoles/μg total RNA, $p < 0.05$). The levels of CK8 in the culture supernatants of these cells, assayed using the established ELISA, were also significantly higher in the NSCLCs than in the SCLCs (310.0 ± 108.0 versus 69.0 ± 18.4 ng/ml, $p < 0.05$). Importantly, the expression level of CK8 mRNA significantly correlated with the measured CK8 protein levels in the culture supernatants of the 17 cell lines ($R = 0.896$, $p < 0.0001$)

CK8 levels in the serum were then determined using this newly established ELISA in 70 consecutive, pathologically-proven lung cancer patients in Kagawa University (male/female, 55/15; median age, 67; performance status, 0/1/2, 16/38/16; histology, adenocarcinoma/squamous cell carcinoma/small cell carcinoma, 25/35/10; disease stage of NSCLC, I/II/III/IV, 10/11/18/21; disease stage of SCLC, limited disease/extensive disease, 4/6). CK8 serum levels were also determined in ten non-smoker normal volunteers. CK8 was detected in the serum of 56 out of 60 patients (93.3%) with NSCLC. The levels of serum CK8 ranged between 0.0 and 595.9 ng/ml. Serum levels of CK8 in NSCLC patients were significantly higher than those in SCLC patients or normal volunteers (86.2 ± 12.1 versus 16.6 ± 5.2 versus 21.2 ± 7.0 ng/ml, $p < 0.05$). The levels of serum CK8 in patients at the advanced stages III and IV were significantly higher than those at the early stages I and II (Fig. 7, A; Figures 7–8. Modified with permission from (Fukunaga et al., 2002)). Similarly, serum CK8 levels of patients with distant metastases were significantly higher than those with no metastases (Fig. 7, B).

A cutoff value of 50 ng/ml was determined based on the highest value observed for serum CK8 in non-smoker volunteers. Fig. 8 demonstrates that NSCLC patients with serum CK8 levels that were higher than this cut-off value showed significantly shortened survival times (Fukunaga et al., 2002).

We demonstrated higher expression levels of CK8 in NSCLC cell lines as well as in culture supernatants, and higher levels of CK8 in the serum of patients with advanced and poor prognosis NSCLC tumors. These results suggest that circulating CK8 may have potential as a novel tumor marker, especially in patients with NSCLC.

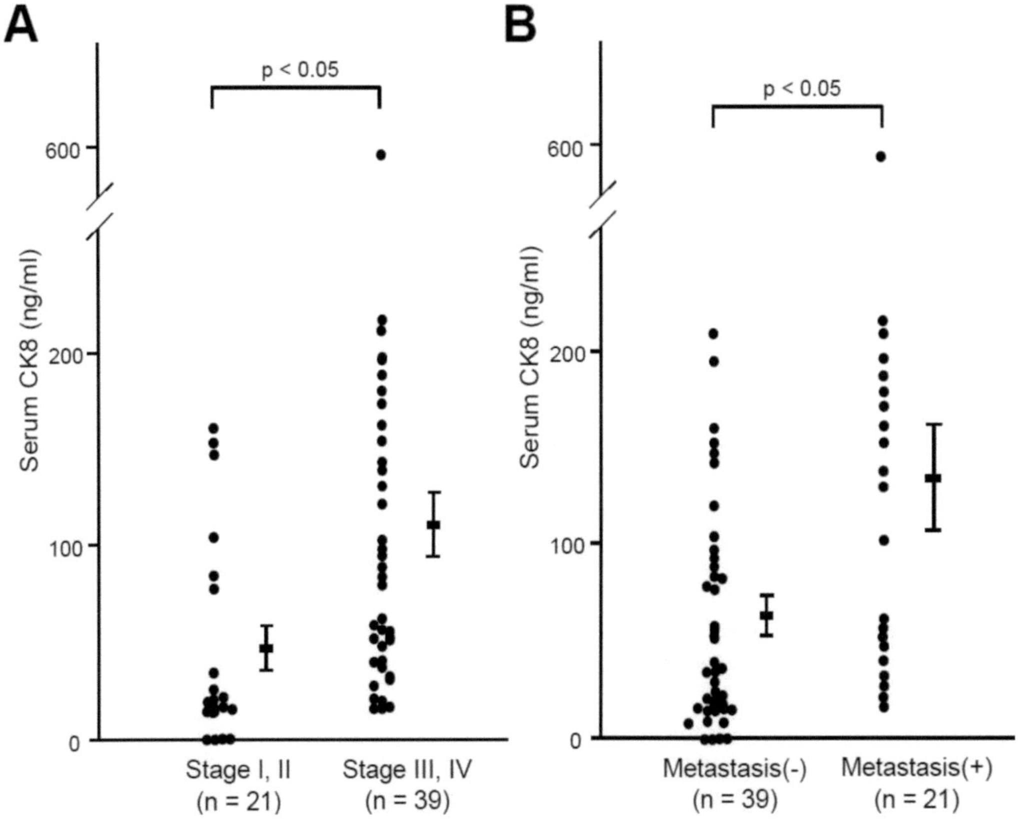

(A) Levels of CK8 in patients with NSCLC at advanced-stages were significantly higher compared with those at earlier stages. (B) Levels of CK8 in patients who had distant metastases of NSCLC were significantly higher compared with those with no distant metastases. To quantify circulating CK8, we established an indirect ELISA using a monoclonal anti-CK8 antibody (M20, purchased from Progen, Heidelberg, Germany). Data are expressed as mean values from duplicate determinations. Mean comparisons of samples were performed using the Mann-Whitney-Wilcoxon test.

Fig. 7. Relationship between tumor progression or distant metastasis and levels of CK8 in the serum of NSCLC patients.

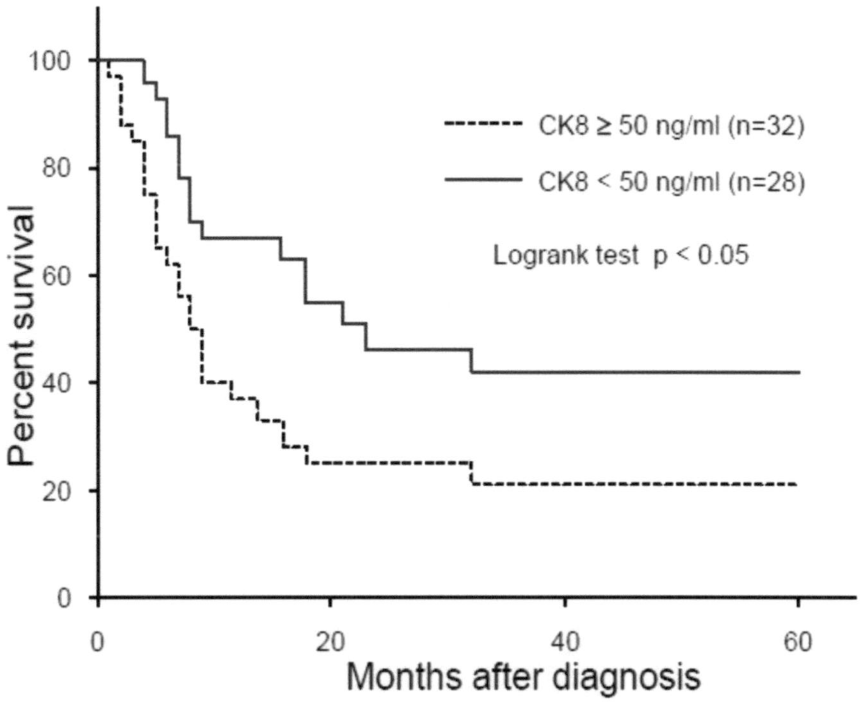

Patients with a CK8 value of 50 ng/ml or higher had a significantly shorter survival time compared with those with lower CK8 values. Survival curves were computed using the Kaplan-Meier method. Mantel's log-rank test was employed to test for equality of survival curves.

Fig. 8. Survival of all patients with NSCLC according to their serum CK8 levels.

5.3 Nature of circulating cytokeratin-related peptides

The nature of circulating CKs in patients with cancer has been widely believed to be CK degradation fragments, which has not been clearly elucidated (Buccheri & Ferrigno, 2001; Pujol et al., 1993; van Dalen, 1996). However, several recent findings may provide some clues to illuminate the characteristics of CK-related molecules in the circulation.

In the cytoplasmic soluble pools, type I-type II CK tetramers appear to be the main components (Alberts et al., 2008; Chou et al., 1993). It sounds plausible that circulating type I and type II CKs may be associated, because CKs intrinsically have a self-bundling potential through their α-helical rod domains, and form primarily heterotetramers in the cytoplasmic soluble pools (Chou et al., 1993; Coulombe & Omary, 2002). Pendleton et al. analyzed serum samples from 24 patients with NSCLC, and detected full length protein of both CK8 and CK18 (Pendleton et al., 1994). In contrast, type I CKs are easily digested by caspases during apoptosis, and these fragments are indeed detected in the circulation as Cyfra 21-1 and as caspase-cleaved CK18 (Buccheri & Ferrigno, 2001; Kramer et al., 2004; Linder et al., 2010; Pujol et al., 1993; Pujol et al., 1996). Unlike type I CKs, type II CKs do not appear to be good caspase substrates. Type II CK8, however, does have potential caspase recognition sequences and effector caspases can cleave CK8 as well as CK18 and CK19, which may be depending on cell types (MacFarlane et al., 2000). Biological significance of caspase recognition sequences in type II CK8 might be illustrated by the presence of aberrantly spliced form of CK8, detected both in lung cancer cell lines and in primary NSCLC tumors. This aberrantly spliced form lacks the caspase cleavage sequence within the linker L12 region, which may confer caspase resistance (Tojo et al., 2003). We also examined circulating CK8 by immunoprecipitation and quantitative immunoblotting from serum samples described above (Fukunaga et al., 2002), and determined that circulating CK8 is mostly (~86%) full length protein (Ishii et al., 2008).

It has not been well understood whether circulating CK-related molecules retain biological functions. Circulation of CK-related polypeptides may not be mere end results of various cellular events and protein processing. For example, phosphorylated type III IF vimentin is released from activated macrophages in response to proinflammatory signaling and is involved in eliminating bacteria and in generating oxidative metabolites, both of which are important functions of activated macropahges (Mor-Vaknin et al., 2003). In case of CKs, we previously reported that antigenically-altered large molecule CK8 contain antigenic epitopes of a tumor marker CA19-9, suggesting that CK8 may function as a carrier protein for CA19-9 (Fujita et al., 1999). As α-helical rod domains are essential for type I-type II heteropolymerization, it is possible that full-length type II CK8 may serve as a binding platform even if circulating type I CKs may partially degrade. Considering the numerous CK-associated proteins, it is also possible that circulating full-length CK8 may form a protein complex with other CK-associated proteins.

6. Issues to be considered when evaluating cytokeratins in tumor cells and in the circulation

Biological relevance of CKs has been intensively studied and myriad of evidence has become accumulated, as discussed in detail in this and other chapters. However, when evaluating these CKs and CK-related products, there are several issues we need to keep in mind (Table 3).

Factors that influence CKs in tumor cells and in the circulation
CK-related molecules in the circulation may reflect: • Expression levels of the individual CKs in the tumor lesions • Total tumor burden • Decay of circulating CK-related products • Production from non-tumorous tissues
CKs in each tumor cell may reflect: • Differentiation status largely depending on cell and/or tissue context • Status of EMT • Invasiveness and metastatic abilities • Cell cycle and cell death

Table 3. Issues to be considered when evaluating CKs in tumor cells and in the circulation

Release of CKs into circulation is a complex multistep process influenced by numerous factors. In tumors expressing CK8/CK18, total amount of CKs likely reflect tumor burden, and also affect the amount of CKs leaking from tumors into extratumoral space, especially into the circulation. Accordingly, the presence of circulating CKs per se does not necessarily reflect characters (e.g. invasiveness and/or metastatic ability) of individual cells. In other words, it is meaningless to evaluate circulating CK-related markers if the original tumors do not express such CKs. Attention need to be paid when evaluating these CK serum markers, because not all lung tumors equally express CK8, CK18 and CK19 (Barak et al., 2004; Karantza, 2011; Linder et al., 2010). Extracellular release of CKs may also be affected by cell deaths (spontaneous or treatment-induced) and cell proliferation. The mechanisms of decay of circulating CK-related products have not been well understood. Apoptotic or necrotic cells are processed by macrophages. The increased turnover of cell proliferation and cell death may overload and subsequently break the clearance mechanisms, which may lead to the accumulation of intracellular components, including CK-related molecules, in the circulation (Linder et al., 2010).

Non-tumorous tissues may become other sources of circulating CKs. Temporal elevations of TPA after surgery for gastric cancer or lung cancer were attributable to tissue repair and physiological cell proliferation as described previously in this chapter (Bauer et al., 1986). Increased serum levels of Cyfra 21-1 were observed in patients with diffuse radiation pneumonitis (inflammation in non-tumorous lung tissues caused by chest radiation therapy), suggesting inflamed lung epithelial tissues as non-cancerous source of circulating CKs (Fujita et al., 2004).

Expression of CKs may reflect differentiation status which seems to depend significantly on cell and/or tissue contexts (Moll et al., 2008; Moll et al., 1982). For example, on various types of epithelial injury, cells may switch from CK8/CK18 to additional CK7 and CK19. This increased CK expression appears to parallel the reduced differentiation (Moll et al., 2008). When tumor cells are acquiring abilities to invade, to resist apoptosis, and to disseminate thorough EMT program, decrement of epithelial markers including CKs and increment of mesenchymal markers including vimentin are often observed (Hanahan & Weinberg, 2011). In contrast to EMT, CKs may also confer aggressiveness to cancer cells as discussed earlier in this chapter.

7. Conclusion

CK8 is the dominant type II IF protein, constituting the primary CK pair with type I CK18, in lung cancer especially in NSCLC. Recent studies have accumulated evidence on understanding roles of CKs as diagnostic markers on tumor pathology, and structural functions of CKs protecting cells from various stress and injuries.

Regulatory functions of CKs seem to be much more multifactorial in terms of cell type- and differentiation stage-dependency as well as numerous interacting factors. At present no definitive roles of CKs in tumor progression have been established, although CKs seem to regulate tumor invasion and metastases positively or negatively by a complex but not fully determined mechanisms. Hopefully future research will solve these questions. Circulating CK-related polypeptides seem to have a potential of clinically meaningful tumor markers. These candidate serum markers await a prospective evaluation in large scale clinical trials.

8. Acknowledgment

We thank Ms. Takimi Tamaki and Ms. Kanako Tejima for their excellent technical assistance. The paper was supported in part by the Japan Society for the Promotion of Science (JSPS) KAKENHI (23501314 and 22790760).

9. References

Alberts, B., et al., (2008). The cytoskeleton. In: *Molecular Bioloby of the Cell,* Alberts, B., et al., pp. 965-1052, Garland Science, Taylor & Francis Group, 978-0-8153-4106-2, Abingdon

Aquilina, R., et al., (1992). [Trials of the diagnostic potentials of TPA in tumorous and nontumorous lung pathologies in 303 cases]. *Minerva Med,* Vol. 83, No. 7-8, (Jul-Aug 1992), pp. 415-9, 0026-4806 (Print) 0026-4806 (Linking)

Barak, V., et al., (2004). Clinical utility of cytokeratins as tumor markers. *Clin Biochem,* Vol. 37, No. 7, (Jul 2004), pp. 529-40, 0009-9120 (Print) 0009-9120 (Linking)

Bauer, T., et al., (1986). Short-term and long-term monitoring of the serum level of TPA after radical resection of gastrointestinal or lung cancer. *Nucl Med Commun,* Vol. 7, No. 2, (Feb 1986), pp. 121-7, 0143-3636 (Print) 0143-3636 (Linking)

Bennink, R., et al., (1999). Serum tissue polypeptide antigen (TPA): monoclonal or polyclonal radio-immunometric assay for the follow-up of bladder cancer. *Anticancer Res,* Vol. 19, No. 4A, (Jul-Aug 1999), pp. 2609-13, 0250-7005 (Print) 0250-7005 (Linking)

Bjorklund, B. & Bjorklund, V., (1983). Specificity and basis of the tissue polypeptide antigen. *Cancer Detect Prev,* Vol. 6, No. 1-2, 1983), pp. 41-50

Brabon, A.C., et al., (1984). A monoclonal antibody to a human breast tumor protein released in response to estrogen. *Cancer Res,* Vol. 44, No. 6, (Jun 1984), pp. 2704-10, 0008-5472 (Print) 0008-5472 (Linking)

Broers, J.L., et al., (1986). Intermediate filament proteins in classic and variant types of small cell lung carcinoma cell lines: a biochemical and immunochemical analysis using a panel of monoclonal and polyclonal antibodies. *J Cell Sci,* Vol. 83, No., (Jul 1986), pp. 37-60, 0021-9533 (Print) 0021-9533 (Linking)

Broers, J.L., et al., (1993). Nuclear A-type lamins are differentially expressed in human lung cancer subtypes. *Am J Pathol,* Vol. 143, No. 1, (Jul 1993), pp. 211-20, 0002-9440 (Print) 0002-9440 (Linking)

Buccheri, G. & Ferrigno, D., (2001). Lung tumor markers of cytokeratin origin: an overview. *Lung Cancer,* Vol. 34 Suppl 2, No., (Dec 2001), pp. S65-9

Buhler, H. & Schaller, G., (2005). Transfection of keratin 18 gene in human breast cancer cells causes induction of adhesion proteins and dramatic regression of malignancy in vitro and in vivo. *Mol Cancer Res,* Vol. 3, No. 7, (Jul 2005), pp. 365-71, 1541-7786 (Print) 1541-7786 (Linking)

Caulin, C., et al., (1997). Caspase cleavage of keratin 18 and reorganization of intermediate filaments during epithelial cell apoptosis. *J Cell Biol,* Vol. 138, No. 6, (Sep 22 1997), pp. 1379-94

Chou, C.F., et al., (1993). A significant soluble keratin fraction in 'simple' epithelial cells. Lack of an apparent phosphorylation and glycosylation role in keratin solubility. *J Cell Sci,* Vol. 105 (Pt 2), No., (Jun 1993), pp. 433-44

Chou, Y.H., et al., (1990). Intermediate filament reorganization during mitosis is mediated by p34cdc2 phosphorylation of vimentin. *Cell,* Vol. 62, No. 6, (Sep 21 1990), pp. 1063-71, 0092-8674 (Print) 0092-8674 (Linking)

Chu, Y.W., et al., (1993). Expression of complete keratin filaments in mouse L cells augments cell migration and invasion. *Proc Natl Acad Sci U S A,* Vol. 90, No. 9, (May 1 1993), pp. 4261-5, 0027-8424 (Print) 0027-8424 (Linking)

Chu, Y.W., et al., (1996). Experimental coexpression of vimentin and keratin intermediate filaments in human melanoma cells augments motility. *Am J Pathol,* Vol. 148, No. 1, (Jan 1996), pp. 63-9, 0002-9440 (Print) 0002-9440 (Linking)

Chu, Y.W., et al., (1997). Selection of invasive and metastatic subpopulations from a human lung adenocarcinoma cell line. *Am J Respir Cell Mol Biol,* Vol. 17, No. 3, (Sep 1997), pp. 353-60, 1044-1549 (Print) 1044-1549 (Linking)

Correale, M., et al., (1994). Clinical profile of a new monoclonal antibody-based immunoassay for tissue polypeptide antigen. *Int J Biol Markers,* Vol. 9, No. 4, (Oct-Dec 1994), pp. 231-8, 0393-6155 (Print) 0393-6155 (Linking)

Coulombe, P.A. & Omary, M.B., (2002). 'Hard' and 'soft' principles defining the structure, function and regulation of keratin intermediate filaments. *Curr Opin Cell Biol,* Vol. 14, No. 1, (Feb 2002), pp. 110-22

Crowe, D.L., et al., (1999). Keratin 19 downregulation by oral squamous cell carcinoma lines increases invasive potential. *J Dent Res,* Vol. 78, No. 6, (Jun 1999), pp. 1256-63, 0022-0345 (Print) 0022-0345 (Linking)

De Petris, L., et al., (2011). Diagnostic and prognostic role of plasma levels of two forms of cytokeratin 18 in patients with non-small-cell lung cancer. *Eur J Cancer,* Vol. 47, No. 1, (Jan 2011), pp. 131-7, 1879-0852 (Electronic) 0959-8049 (Linking)

Dohmoto, K., et al., (2000). Mechanisms of the release of CYFRA21-1 in human lung cancer cell lines. *Lung Cancer,* Vol. 30, No. 1, (Oct 2000), pp. 55-63

Dohmoto, K., et al., (2001). The role of caspase 3 in producing cytokeratin 19 fragment (CYFRA21-1) in human lung cancer cell lines. *Int J Cancer,* Vol. 91, No. 4, (Feb 15 2001), pp. 468-73

Eriksson, J.E., et al., (2004). Specific in vivo phosphorylation sites determine the assembly dynamics of vimentin intermediate filaments. *J Cell Sci,* Vol. 117, No. Pt 6, (Feb 29 2004), pp. 919-32, 0021-9533 (Print) 0021-9533 (Linking)

Fisher, D.Z., et al., (1986). cDNA sequencing of nuclear lamins A and C reveals primary and secondary structural homology to intermediate filament proteins. *Proc Natl Acad Sci U S A,* Vol. 83, No. 17, (Sep 1986), pp. 6450-4, 0027-8424 (Print) 0027-8424 (Linking)

Fuchs, E. & Karakesisoglou, I., (2001). Bridging cytoskeletal intersections. *Genes Dev,* Vol. 15, No. 1, (Jan 1 2001), pp. 1-14, 0890-9369 (Print) 0890-9369 (Linking)

Fujita, J., et al., (1999). Detection of large molecular weight cytokeratin 8 as carrier protein of CA19-9 in non-small-cell lung cancer cell lines. *Br J Cancer,* Vol. 81, No. 5, (Nov 1999), pp. 769-73

Fujita, J., et al., (2001). The point mutation in the promoter region and the single nucleotide polymorphism in exon 1 of the cytokeratin 19 gene in human lung cancer cell lines. *Lung Cancer,* Vol. 34, No. 3, (Dec 2001), pp. 387-94, 0169-5002 (Print) 0169-5002 (Linking)

Fujita, J., et al., (2004). Elevation of cytokeratin 19 fragment (CYFRA 21-1) in serum of patients with radiation pneumonitis: possible marker of epithelial cell damage.

Respir Med, Vol. 98, No. 4, (Apr 2004), pp. 294-300, 0954-6111 (Print) 0954-6111 (Linking)

Fukunaga, Y., et al., (2002). Expression of cytokeratin 8 in lung cancer cell lines and measurement of serum cytokeratin 8 in lung cancer patients. *Lung Cancer,* Vol. 38, No. 1, (Oct 2002), pp. 31-8

Fuxe, J., et al., (2010). Transcriptional crosstalk between TGF-beta and stem cell pathways in tumor cell invasion: role of EMT promoting Smad complexes. *Cell Cycle,* Vol. 9, No. 12, (Jun 15 2010), pp. 2363-74, 1551-4005 (Electronic) 1551-4005 (Linking)

Gion, M., et al., (2000). Quantitative measurement of soluble cytokeratin fragments in tissue cytosol of 599 node negative breast cancer patients: a prognostic marker possibly associated with apoptosis. *Breast Cancer Res Treat,* Vol. 59, No. 3, (Feb 2000), pp. 211-21, 0167-6806 (Print) 0167-6806 (Linking)

Giovanella, L., et al., (1995). Tissue polypeptide specific antigen (tps) and cytokeratin 19 fragment (CYFRA 21.1) immunoradiometric assay in non small cell lung cancer evaluation. *Q J Nucl Med,* Vol. 39, No. 4, (Dec 1995), pp. 285-9, 1125-0135 (Print) 1125-0135 (Linking)

Goldstraw, P., et al., (2007). The IASLC Lung Cancer Staging Project: proposals for the revision of the TNM stage groupings in the forthcoming (seventh) edition of the TNM Classification of malignant tumours. *J Thorac Oncol,* Vol. 2, No. 8, (Aug 2007), pp. 706-14, 1556-1380 (Electronic) 1556-0864 (Linking)

Hanahan, D. & Weinberg, R.A., (2011). Hallmarks of cancer: the next generation. *Cell,* Vol. 144, No. 5, (Mar 4 2011), pp. 646-74, 1097-4172 (Electronic) 0092-8674 (Linking)

Hendrix, M.J., et al., (1992). Coexpression of vimentin and keratins by human melanoma tumor cells: correlation with invasive and metastatic potential. *J Natl Cancer Inst,* Vol. 84, No. 3, (Feb 5 1992), pp. 165-74, 0027-8874 (Print) 0027-8874 (Linking)

Hutchison, C.J., (2002). Lamins: building blocks or regulators of gene expression? *Nat Rev Mol Cell Biol,* Vol. 3, No. 11, (Nov 2002), pp. 848-58, 1471-0072 (Print) 1471-0072 (Linking)

Ishii, T., et al., (2008). Full-length cytokeratin 8 is released and circulates in patients with non-small cell lung cancer. *Tumour Biol,* Vol. 29, No. 1, 2008), pp. 57-62, 1423-0380 (Electronic) 1010-4283 (Linking)

Jemal, A., et al., (2011). Global cancer statistics. *CA Cancer J Clin,* Vol. 61, No. 2, (Mar-Apr 2011), pp. 69-90, 1542-4863 (Electronic) 0007-9235 (Linking)

Kanaji, N., et al., (2007). Compensation of type I and type II cytokeratin pools in lung cancer. *Lung Cancer,* Vol. 55, No. 3, (Mar 2007), pp. 295-302, 0169-5002 (Print) 0169-5002 (Linking)

Kanaji, N., et al., (2011). Cytokeratins negatively regulate the invasive potential of lung cancer cell lines. *Oncol Rep,* Vol. 26, No. 4, (Oct 2011), pp. 763-8, 1791-2431 (Electronic) 1021-335X (Linking)

Karantza, V., (2011). Keratins in health and cancer: more than mere epithelial cell markers. *Oncogene,* Vol. 30, No. 2, (Jan 13 2011), pp. 127-38, 1476-5594 (Electronic) 0950-9232 (Linking)

Kasai, H., et al., (2005). TGF-beta1 induces human alveolar epithelial to mesenchymal cell transition (EMT). *Respir Res,* Vol. 6, No., 2005), pp. 56, 1465-993X (Electronic) 1465-9921 (Linking)

Kim, K.H., et al., (1984). Expression of unusually large keratins during terminal differentiation: balance of type I and type II keratins is not disrupted. *J Cell Biol,* Vol. 99, No. 5, (Nov 1984), pp. 1872-7, 0021-9525 (Print) 0021-9525 (Linking)

Knosel, T., et al., (2006). Cytokeratin profiles identify diagnostic signatures in colorectal cancer using multiplex analysis of tissue microarrays. *Cell Oncol,* Vol. 28, No. 4, 2006), pp. 167-75, 1570-5870 (Print) 1570-5870 (Linking)

Koelink, P.J., et al., (2009). Circulating cell death products predict clinical outcome of colorectal cancer patients. *BMC Cancer,* Vol. 9, No., 2009), pp. 88, 1471-2407 (Electronic) 1471-2407 (Linking)

Kouklis, P.D., et al., (1994). Making a connection: direct binding between keratin intermediate filaments and desmosomal proteins. *J Cell Biol,* Vol. 127, No. 4, (Nov 1994), pp. 1049-60, 0021-9525 (Print) 0021-9525 (Linking)

Kramer, G., et al., (2004). Differentiation between cell death modes using measurements of different soluble forms of extracellular cytokeratin 18. *Cancer Res,* Vol. 64, No. 5, (Mar 1 2004), pp. 1751-6

Ku, N.O., et al., (2002). Keratin binding to 14-3-3 proteins modulates keratin filaments and hepatocyte mitotic progression. *Proc Natl Acad Sci U S A,* Vol. 99, No. 7, (Apr 2 2002), pp. 4373-8, 0027-8424 (Print) 0027-8424 (Linking)

Li, Q.Q., et al., (2009). Twist1-mediated adriamycin-induced epithelial-mesenchymal transition relates to multidrug resistance and invasive potential in breast cancer cells. *Clin Cancer Res,* Vol. 15, No. 8, (Apr 15 2009), pp. 2657-65, 1078-0432 (Print) 1078-0432 (Linking)

Liao, J. & Omary, M.B., (1996). 14-3-3 proteins associate with phosphorylated simple epithelial keratins during cell cycle progression and act as a solubility cofactor. *J Cell Biol,* Vol. 133, No. 2, (Apr 1996), pp. 345-57, 0021-9525 (Print) 0021-9525 (Linking)

Linder, S., et al., (2010). Utilization of cytokeratin-based biomarkers for pharmacodynamic studies. *Expert Rev Mol Diagn,* Vol. 10, No. 3, (Apr 2010), pp. 353-9, 1744-8352 (Electronic) 1473-7159 (Linking)

MacFarlane, M., et al., (2000). Active caspases and cleaved cytokeratins are sequestered into cytoplasmic inclusions in TRAIL-induced apoptosis. *J Cell Biol,* Vol. 148, No. 6, (Mar 20 2000), pp. 1239-54

McKeon, F.D., et al., (1986). Homologies in both primary and secondary structure between nuclear envelope and intermediate filament proteins. *Nature,* Vol. 319, No. 6053, (Feb 6-12 1986), pp. 463-8, 0028-0836 (Print) 0028-0836 (Linking)

Mellerick, D.M., et al., (1990). On the nature of serological tissue polypeptide antigen (TPA); monoclonal keratin 8, 18, and 19 antibodies react differently with TPA prepared from human cultured carcinoma cells and TPA in human serum. *Oncogene,* Vol. 5, No. 7, (Jul 1990), pp. 1007-17, 0950-9232 (Print) 0950-9232 (Linking)

Moll, R., et al., (2008). The human keratins: biology and pathology. *Histochem Cell Biol,* Vol. 129, No. 6, (Jun 2008), pp. 705-33, 0948-6143 (Print) 0948-6143 (Linking)

Moll, R., et al., (1982). The catalog of human cytokeratins: patterns of expression in normal epithelia, tumors and cultured cells. *Cell,* Vol. 31, No. 1, (Nov 1982), pp. 11-24

Mor-Vaknin, N., et al., (2003). Vimentin is secreted by activated macrophages. *Nat Cell Biol,* Vol. 5, No. 1, (Jan 2003), pp. 59-63

NCCN.org. (July 1, 2011). NCCN Clinical Practice Guidelines in Oncoloty Non-Small Cell Lung Cancer, In: *World Wide Web Sites,* July 31, 2011, Available from: <http://www.nccn.org/professionals/physician_gls/pdf/nscl.pdf>

Nicolini, A., et al., (1995). Usefulness of CEA, TPA, GICA, CA 72.4, and CA 195 in the Diagnosis of primary colorectal cancer and at its relapse. *Cancer Detect Prev,* Vol. 19, No. 2, 1995), pp. 183-95, 0361-090X (Print) 0361-090X (Linking)

Nisman, B., et al., (1998). Evaluation of tissue polypeptide specific antigen, CYFRA 21-1, and carcinoembryonic antigen in nonsmall cell lung carcinoma: does the combined use of cytokeratin markers give any additional information? *Cancer,* Vol. 82, No. 10, (May 15 1998), pp. 1850-9, 0008-543X (Print) 0008-543X (Linking)

Omary, M.B., et al., (2006). "Heads and tails" of intermediate filament phosphorylation: multiple sites and functional insights. *Trends Biochem Sci,* Vol. 31, No. 7, (Jul 2006), pp. 383-94, 0968-0004 (Print) 0968-0004 (Linking)

Oshima, R.G., (2002). Apoptosis and keratin intermediate filaments. *Cell Death Differ,* Vol. 9, No. 5, (May 2002), pp. 486-92

Pendleton, N., et al., (1994). Simple cytokeratins in the serum of patients with lung cancer: relationship to cell death. *Eur J Cancer,* Vol. 30A, No. 1, 1994), pp. 93-6

Plebani, M., et al., (1995). Clinical evaluation of seven tumour markers in lung cancer diagnosis: can any combination improve the results? *Br J Cancer,* Vol. 72, No. 1, (Jul 1995), pp. 170-3, 0007-0920 (Print) 0007-0920 (Linking)

Pujol, J.L., et al., (1994). Clinical evaluation of serum tissue polypeptide-specific antigen (TPS) in non-small cell lung cancer. *Eur J Cancer,* Vol. 30A, No. 12, 1994), pp. 1768-74, 0959-8049 (Print) 0959-8049 (Linking)

Pujol, J.L., et al., (1993). Serum fragment of cytokeratin subunit 19 measured by CYFRA 21-1 immunoradiometric assay as a marker of lung cancer. *Cancer Res,* Vol. 53, No. 1, (Jan 1 1993), pp. 61-6

Pujol, J.L., et al., (1996). Cytokeratins as serum markers in lung cancer: a comparison of CYFRA 21-1 and TPS. *Am J Respir Crit Care Med,* Vol. 154, No. 3 Pt 1, (Sep 1996), pp. 725-33, 1073-449X (Print) 1073-449X (Linking)

Quinlan, R.A., et al., (1985). Patterns of expression and organization of cytokeratin intermediate filaments. *Ann N Y Acad Sci,* Vol. 455, No., 1985), pp. 282-306

Rieger-Christ, K.M., et al., (2005). Restoration of plakoglobin expression in bladder carcinoma cell lines suppresses cell migration and tumorigenic potential. *Br J Cancer,* Vol. 92, No. 12, (Jun 20 2005), pp. 2153-9, 0007-0920 (Print) 0007-0920 (Linking)

Rodriguez, E. & Lilenbaum, R.C., (2010). Small cell lung cancer: past, present, and future. *Curr Oncol Rep,* Vol. 12, No. 5, (Sep 2010), pp. 327-34, 1534-6269 (Electronic) 1523-3790 (Linking)

Rosati, G., et al., (2000). Use of tumor markers in the management of head and neck cancer. *Int J Biol Markers,* Vol. 15, No. 2, (Apr-Jun 2000), pp. 179-83, 0393-6155 (Print) 0393-6155 (Linking)

Satelli, A. & Li, S., (2011). Vimentin in cancer and its potential as a molecular target for cancer therapy. *Cell Mol Life Sci,* Vol. 68, No. 18, (Sep 2011), pp. 3033-46, 1420-9071 (Electronic) 1420-682X (Linking)

Schaller, G., et al., (1996). Elevated keratin 18 protein expression indicates a favorable prognosis in patients with breast cancer. *Clin Cancer Res,* Vol. 2, No. 11, (Nov 1996), pp. 1879-85, 1078-0432 (Print) 1078-0432 (Linking)

Sheard, M.A., et al., (2002). Release of cytokeratin-18 and -19 fragments (TPS and CYFRA 21-1) into the extracellular space during apoptosis. *J Cell Biochem,* Vol. 85, No. 4, 2002), pp. 670-7

Shih, J.Y. & Yang, P.C., (2011). The EMT regulator slug and lung carcinogenesis. *Carcinogenesis,* Vol., No., (Jun 30 2011), pp., 1460-2180 (Electronic) 0143-3334 (Linking)

Sihag, R.K., et al., (2007). Role of phosphorylation on the structural dynamics and function of types III and IV intermediate filaments. *Exp Cell Res,* Vol. 313, No. 10, (Jun 10 2007), pp. 2098-109, 0014-4827 (Print) 0014-4827 (Linking)

Simon, G.R. & Turrisi, A., (2007). Management of small cell lung cancer: ACCP evidence-based clinical practice guidelines (2nd edition). *Chest,* Vol. 132, No. 3 Suppl, (Sep 2007), pp. 324S-339S, 0012-3692 (Print) 0012-3692 (Linking)

Smith, E.A. & Fuchs, E., (1998). Defining the interactions between intermediate filaments and desmosomes. *J Cell Biol,* Vol. 141, No. 5, (Jun 1 1998), pp. 1229-41, 0021-9525 (Print) 0021-9525 (Linking)

Soletormos, G., et al., (2004). Monitoring different stages of breast cancer using tumour markers CA 15-3, CEA and TPA. *Eur J Cancer,* Vol. 40, No. 4, (Mar 2004), pp. 481-6, 0959-8049 (Print) 0959-8049 (Linking)

South, A.P., et al., (2003). Lack of plakophilin 1 increases keratinocyte migration and reduces desmosome stability. *J Cell Sci,* Vol. 116, No. Pt 16, (Aug 15 2003), pp. 3303-14, 0021-9533 (Print) 0021-9533 (Linking)

Steinert, P.M., et al., (1993). Conservation of the structure of keratin intermediate filaments: molecular mechanism by which different keratin molecules integrate into preexisting keratin intermediate filaments during differentiation. *Biochemistry,* Vol. 32, No. 38, (Sep 28 1993), pp. 10046-56, 0006-2960 (Print) 0006-2960 (Linking)

Takeyama, Y., et al., (2010). Knockdown of ZEB1, a master epithelial-to-mesenchymal transition (EMT) gene, suppresses anchorage-independent cell growth of lung cancer cells. *Cancer Lett,* Vol. 296, No. 2, (Oct 28 2010), pp. 216-24, 1872-7980 (Electronic) 0304-3835 (Linking)

Tinnemans, M.M., et al., (1995). Alterations in cytoskeletal and nuclear matrix-associated proteins during apoptosis. *Eur J Cell Biol,* Vol. 68, No. 1, (Sep 1995), pp. 35-46, 0171-9335 (Print) 0171-9335 (Linking)

Tojo, Y., et al., (2003). Aberrant messenger RNA splicing of the cytokeratin 8 in lung cancer. *Lung Cancer,* Vol. 42, No. 2, (Nov 2003), pp. 153-61, 0169-5002 (Print) 0169-5002 (Linking)

Ueda, Y., et al., (1999). Expression of cytokeratin 19 mRNA in human lung cancer cell lines. *Int J Cancer,* Vol. 81, No. 6, (Jun 11 1999), pp. 939-43

van Dalen, A., (1996). Significance of cytokeratin markers TPA, TPA (cyk), TPS and CYFRA 21.1 in metastatic disease. *Anticancer Res,* Vol. 16, No. 4B, (Jul-Aug 1996), pp. 2345-9

van der Gaast, A., et al., (1994). Prognostic significance of tissue polypeptide-specific antigen (TPS) in patients with advanced non-small cell lung cancer. *Eur J Cancer,* Vol. 30A, No. 12, 1994), pp. 1783-6, 0959-8049 (Print) 0959-8049 (Linking)

Woelfle, U., et al., (2004). Down-regulated expression of cytokeratin 18 promotes progression of human breast cancer. *Clin Cancer Res,* Vol. 10, No. 8, (Apr 15 2004), pp. 2670-4, 1078-0432 (Print) 1078-0432 (Linking)

Yamashiro, Y., et al., (2010). Ectopic coexpression of keratin 8 and 18 promotes invasion of transformed keratinocytes and is induced in patients with cutaneous squamous cell carcinoma. *Biochem Biophys Res Commun,* Vol. 399, No. 3, (Aug 27 2010), pp. 365-72, 1090-2104 (Electronic) 0006-291X (Linking)

Yee, D.S., et al., (2010). The Wnt inhibitory factor 1 restoration in prostate cancer cells was associated with reduced tumor growth, decreased capacity of cell migration and invasion and a reversal of epithelial to mesenchymal transition. *Mol Cancer,* Vol. 9, No., 2010), pp. 162, 1476-4598 (Electronic) 1476-4598 (Linking)

Yen, T.C., et al., (1998). A study of a new tumour marker, CYFRA 21-1, in squamous cell carcinoma of the head and neck, and comparison with squamous cell carcinoma antigen. *Clin Otolaryngol Allied Sci,* Vol. 23, No. 1, (Feb 1998), pp. 82-6, 0307-7772 (Print) 0307-7772 (Linking)

Youlden, D.R., et al., (2008). The International Epidemiology of Lung Cancer: geographical distribution and secular trends. *J Thorac Oncol,* Vol. 3, No. 8, (Aug 2008), pp. 819-31, 1556-1380 (Electronic) 1556-0864 (Linking)

Part 3

Cytokeratins as Markers of Tumor Dissemination and Response

6

Cytokeratin 18 (CK18) and CK18 Fragments for Detection of Minimal Residual Disease in Colon Cancer Patients

Ulrike Olszewski-Hamilton, Veronika Buxhofer-Ausch, Christoph Ausch and Gerhard Hamilton*
Ludwig Boltzmann Cluster of Translational Oncology, Vienna, Austria

1. Introduction

Despite advances in therapeutic approaches for patients with colorectal cancer (CRC), approximately 20-45% of those who undergo apparently curative surgery subsequently develop local or distant tumor recurrence (Harrison & Benziger, 2011). The liver constitutes the preferred metastatic site in approximately 30% of cases. According to the TNM staging system, a stage-specific 5-year survival rate of approximately 93% has to be expected for stage I, 72-84% for stage II, 44-83% for stage III and 8% for stage IV colon cancer (O'Connell et al., 2004). An early identification of patients at risk of developing metastatic disease after surgery would be of great importance for improving the clinical outcome. Currently, there are no reliable methods to identify patients who are at increased risk of relapse and in need of adjuvant chemotherapy. Aggressive postoperative treatment with cytotoxic drugs without certain indication leads to overtreatment of patients and severe side effects. Appropriate biomarkers for the identification of CRC patients at high risk for recurrence and/or poor prognosis are required to facilitate individually tailored therapy (Gangadhar et al., 2010).

1.1 Biomarkers and CRC

In general, an eligible biomarker in reference to chemotherapy is a characteristic that is objectively measured and evaluated as an indicator of response. A range of assays, including immunohistochemistry, gene analysis, gene and protein expression assessments and detection of single nucleotide polymorphisms (SNPs) have served to identify biomarkers in recent years (Saijo, 2011). Response rates to anticancer drugs applied in CRC may be as low as approximately 20% and, therefore, it is of great importance to identify patients most likely to benefit from a specific agent. For example, biomarkers such as expression of HER2 for breast cancer or EGFR mutation for lung cancer and KRAS mutation in CRC aid in selection of drug-sensitive patients. Personalized CRC care has improved patient outcome significantly over the last decades in both the adjuvant and metastatic

---

* Corresponding Author

settings (Catenacci et al., 2011). Microarray-based gene expression profiling has been frequently used to formulate prognostic signatures and, to a lesser degree, predictive signatures in CRC; however, common problems associated with these markers are clinical study design, reproducibility and interpretation of the results (Van Schaeybroeck et al., 2011).

1.2 CRC and disseminated tumor cells (DTCs)

Approximately 50% of CRC patients undergoing curative resection die from metastatic disease within 5 years and the relapse rate is 30% even in lymph node-negative patients (Iddings & Bilchik, 2007). Appearance of disseminated tumor cells (DTCs) in cancer patients may precede the occurrence of detectable metastases and, thus, may be used to adapt the aggressiveness of therapeutic regimens (Lugo et al., 2003; Pantel & Alix-Panabières, 2010). First evidence for such a role of bone marrow DTCs (BM-DTCs) or circulating tumor cells (CTCs), respectively, was obtained for breast cancer, where BM-positive patients had an approximately twofold increased risk of relapse within ten years (Braun et al., 2000). However, the situation is less clear for other solid tumors like CRC (Thorsteinsson & Jess, 2011). Both solitary cells and micrometastases may remain in "dormancy" for years, being cell cycle arrested and not undergoing apoptosis (Luzzi et al., 1998). Cancer cells that left the primary tumor can seed metastases in distant organs, which is thought to be a unidirectional process. However, in a process that is called "tumor self-seeding" CTCs can also colonize their tumor of origin (Kim et al., 2009).

As further discussed below, analysis of cytokeratins (CKs), either by RT-PCR, immunohistochemistry or quantification of soluble CK protein fragments released by tumor cells, is the mainstay of the detection of DTCs. Studies indicate that BM is a common homing organ and serves as reservoir for DTCs derived from various primary sites including tumors of the breast, prostate, lung and colon (Pantel & Alix-Panabières, 2010). However, peripheral blood analyses are obviously more convenient for patients than invasive BM sampling.

1.3 CKs as marker of epithelial tumor cells

Antibodies directed to CKs, that are members of the intermediate filament (IF) proteins, are useful tools particularly in the diagnostics of carcinomas (Barak et al., 2004; Karantza, 2011). These proteins protect epithelial cells from mechanical and non-mechanical stressors (Coulombe & Omary, 2002). At present, more than 20 different CKs have been identified, of which CKs 8, 18, and 19 are the most abundant in simple epithelial cells and carcinomas of the breast, prostate, lung, colon, ovary, among others (Moll et al., 1982; Bragulla & Homberger, 2009). Low molecular weight acidic type I CKs, such as CK18, are normally complexed with high molecular weight basic or neutral type II CKs, such as CK8. The bulk of cellular CKs are part of the IF system and mostly insoluble at physiological salt concentrations until they are cleaved to yield soluble fragments. CKs are in use for the detection of epithelial cancer cells in BM with the help of pan-CK antibodies directed to the CKs 8, 18, 19 and, furthermore, these proteins seem to be of functional importance for BM-DTCs. Alix-Panabieres et al. demonstrated that full-length CK19 was shed by viable epithelial breast tumor cells and that such cells might constitute a biologically active subset of breast cancer cells with highly metastatic properties (Alix-Panabieres et al., 2009).

The production of soluble CK fragments may be triggered by hypoxia that has resulted in network disassembly and CK8/CK18 degradation (Na et al., 2010). Similarly, the keratin cytoskeleton in mammary epithelial cells disintegrates under metabolic stress of glucose and oxygen deprivation, which mimicks the tumor microenvironment (Nelson et al., 2004) Phosphorylation of CKs regulates their distribution into an insoluble filamentous cytoskeletal fraction and a soluble cytosolic hyperphosphorylated pool (Omary et al., 2006) and plays a role in CK ubiquitination and turnover by the proteasome (Ku & Omary, 2000; Jaitovich et al., 2008) and, likely, by autophagy (Kongara et al., 2010). CKs released from proliferating or necrotic/apoptotic cells are useful markers for prediction of tumor progression/recurrence or response to therapy (Linder, 2007). The three most applied CK markers for the assessment of cell activity used in the clinic are tissue polypeptide antigen (TPA), tissue polypeptide-specific antigen (TPS) and CYFRA 21-1. The broad spectrum TPA test measures CKs 8, 18, and 19 concentrations, while TPS and CYFRA 21-1 assays are more specific and determine CK18 and CK 19 levels, respectively (Linder, 2007). More recently, the ratio of caspase-cleaved (M30) to total CK18 (M65), which can be assessed in the serum or plasma using commercially available enzyme-linked immunosorbent assay (ELISA) kits, has been evaluated as a biomarker for monitoring therapy efficacy in carcinoma patients (Linder et al., 2010).

2. Assessment of DTCs in CRC

The prognosis of colon cancer patients is largely determined by the occurrence of systemic disease (Negin & Cohen, 2010). In patients with primary tumors relapse is mainly due to clinically occult micrometastasis that exists in secondary organs already at first presentation, but is not detectable with imaging procedures currently used (Riethdorf et al., 2008). Sensitive and specific immunocytochemical and molecular tests enable the assessment and characterization of DTCs at the single cell level in BM, which constitutes the common homing site of DTCs. Although many assays were developed to prove CTCs, two main approaches that are used involve either cytology based on immunocytochemical staining or polymerase chain reaction (PCR) analysis (Cristofanilli et al., 2007). Employing the US Food and Drug Administration (FDA)-approved Cellsearch® system, the value of CTCs as a predictive marker for survival was substantiated in metastatic breast cancer and CRC (Paterlini-Brechot et al., 2007). Still, there is an urgent need for standardized methods because of the high variability of results in the detection of DTCs and CTCs, respectively.

2.1 Detection of DTCs by RT-PCR

The detection of CTCs can be very difficult with as few as one CTC in 100 million leukocytes in peripheral blood and, thus, highly sensitive methods like PCR are employed to detect tumor-specific DNA or RNA. Since RNA is unstable and therefore disappears quickly from the blood after cell death, presence of RNA must be due to the occurence of viable tumor cells (Mostert et al., 2009). The RNA markers commonly used in CRC are carcinoembryonic antigen (CEA), CK19 and CK20 (Sergeant et al., 2008). The advantage of RT-PCR is a higher sensitivity compared to immunocytochemical techniques. Unfortunately, the specificity of RT-PCR is hampered by high numbers of false-positive results either due to contamination or target genes expressed in other nonmalignant cells. Novaes et al. demonstrated that mononuclear cells from peripheral blood of healthy donors express CK19 in RT-PCR assays (Novaes et al., 1997). Furthermore, both CEA and CK20 transcripts are elevated in patients with inflammatory diseases (Dandachi et al., 2005). Another important limitation of PCR-based methods is that CTCs cannot be isolated for further analysis. Nevertheless, Allen-Mersh et al. demonstrated that poor disease-free survival (DFS) was associated with the occurrence of CEA or CK20 24 hrs postoperatively using RT-PCR on blood samples from 147 CRC patients with TNM-stage I-III tumors (Allen-Mersh et al., 2007). In another study, four RNA markers including human telomerase reverse transcriptase (hTERT), CK19, CK20 and CEA mRNA were used to detect CTCs in stages II and III CRC patients who underwent curative resection to determine the significance of CTCs in prediction of early relapse (Lu et al., 2011). The presence of persistent postoperative CTCs was proved as independent predictor for early recurrence (hazard ratio: 11.04) and correlated with a poorer DFS and overall survival (OS). CK20 is a commonly used RT-PCR marker in analysis of BM from CRC patients; however, the number of investigated patients was larger than 100 with DTC detection rates of 11-35% only in 3 out of 10 studies. Two groups reported no association to survival in metastatic patients, whereas four groups found a correlation between the presence of CK20 transcripts and worse OS (Koch et al., 2006).

Rahbari et al. also found postoperative tumor cell detection can predict poor recurrence-free survival in curatively resected CRC patients in a metaanalysis (Rahbari et al., 2010). The included studies reported postoperative detection rates of 22-57% DTCs in CRC with RT-PCR. However, application of the RT-PCR approach is hampered by an absence of an international standard on choice of markers, enrichment procedures and laboratory techniques. Nevertheless, combining the TNM staging system and proof of CTCs could aid in decision-making as to which patients should be offered adjuvant chemotherapy.

2.2 Detection of DTCs by immunohistochemical methods

Immunohistochemistry utilizes labeled monoclonal antibodies directed against epithelial or tumor-associated antigens and automated digital microscopy or flow cytometry to isolate and count CTCs (Alix-Panabieres et al., 2008; Pantel et al., 2009; Allen & Keeney, 2010). This method allows identification of intact tumor cells occurring in the periphery for further characterization (Smirnov et al., 2005; Cohen et al., 2006). Most studies describing immunocytochemistry for the detection of DTCs in CRC patients either used the monoclonal antibody CK2 against CK18 or the pan-cytokeratin antibody A45-B/B3, while few studies employed a cocktail of several antibodies against different epithelial antigens including CKs. The DTC detection rate in studies with CK2 was 16-32%, whereas it was clearly higher in investigations using the A45-B/B3 antibody (24-55%). This difference might probably be due to a potential downregulation or loss of CK18 expression on DTCs (Pantel et al., 1994). Both antibodies rarely detect CK-positive cells in BM of noncancer control patients (0-5.5%). The largest study so far conducted by Flatmark et al. included 275 CRC patients and 206 noncancer control patients (Flatmark et al., 2011). An immunomagnetic bead enrichment system capturing BM-DTCs by the antibody MOC31 directed against epithelial cell adhesion molecule (EpCAM) was applied and 17% of the patients showed presence of DTCs, whereas only 1.5% of control samples were positive. However, the BM status did not correlate significantly with disease stage or other clinical parameters, a finding we confirmed in a small series of patients (Buxhofer-Ausch et al., 2009). In conclusion, several studies were carried out to elucidate the clinical relevance of DTCs in CRC. These studies, however, present a very heterogeneous picture differing in patient groups, sample sizes, follow-up times, staining methods and target antigens, all of which probably contributed to the observed variation in DTC detection rates and association to clinical parameters (Riethdorf et al., 2008).

For the analysis of CTCs an automated microscopic system including an immunomagnetic tumor cell enrichment step was developed (Miller et al., 2010). This CellSearch System (Veridex LLC, Raritan, NJ) gained approval for metastatic breast cancer from the FDA in 2004 and is now also accepted for metastatic prostate and colorectal cancer. In this detection method CTCs must feature: a round to oval shape by light scatter, an evident nucleus by DAPI staining, EpCAM positivity and $CK8^+$, $CK18^+$, $CK19^+$ and $CD45^-$ by immunofluorescence (Allard et al., 2004). The sensitivity of approaches using EpCAM might be limited by the fact that EpCAM-negative CTCs would not be detected, which would lead to false-negative results. Rao et al. demonstrated that the expression of EpCAM on CTCs was approximately tenfold lower than on primary and metastatic tissues (Rao et al., 2005). The CellSearch CTC detection system was combined with a monoclonal antibody (M30) targeting a neoepitope disclosed by caspase cleavage at CK18 in early apoptosis (Rossi et al., 2010). M30-positive CTC could be detected in >70% of CTC-positive carcinoma patients, which were free from both chemotherapy and radiologic treatments. The fraction of M30-positive CTC varied from 50% to 80%, depending on the histotype.

In a study by Sastre et al., CTCs were detected in 34 of 94 patients (Sastre et al., 2008). Only tumor stage correlated with positive CTCs (20.7% in stage II, 24.1% in stage III and 60.7% in stage IV). Cohen et al. demonstrated that the CTC level at baseline and follow-up is an independent prognostic factor in metastatic CRC. Patients were divided into unfavorable and favorable prognostic groups by their CTC levels of ≥3 or <3 CTCs/7.5 ml blood, respectively. PFS as well as OS was shorter for unfavorable compared with favorable baseline CTC patients (Cohen et al., 2009). Approximately one quarter of patients with metastatic disease thereby categorized in this poor prognosis group (Negin & Cohen, 2010). In a similar study by Tol et al. the CTC count before and during treatment with chemotherapy plus targeted agents independently predicted PFS and OS in advanced CRC patients (Tol et al., 2010). A metaanalysis of available studies to assess whether the detection of tumor cells in the blood and BM of patients diagnosed with primary CRC can be used as a prognostic factor included a total of 36 reports, comprising 3094 patients (Rahbari et al., 2010). Pooled analyses that combined all sampling sites showed an association of the detection of tumor cells with poor DFS (hazard ration: 3.24) and OS (hazard ratio: 2.28). Now there is compelling evidence that CTCs predict clinical response in metastatic CRC (Allen & El-Deiry, 2010).

Although the presence of CTCs can be a strong marker of poor prognosis in patients with metastatic disease, the prognostic role of CTCs in nonmetastatic CRC (TNM stages I-III) is less clear (Thorsteinsson & Jess, 2011a). By using the CellSearch method to detect CTCs from blood samples taken 4-12 weeks after apparently curative surgery, Maestro et al. found >2 CTCs/7.5 ml blood in 25 of 164 patients with localized CRC (Maestro et al., 2009). CTCs were detected with the CellSearch system preoperatively in one out of 20 patients with TNM stages I-III, and none of the four different postoperative blood samples had CTC levels above the cut-off value of ≥2 CTCs/7.5 ml blood (Thorsteinsson et al., 2011b). The presence of CTCs at least 24 hrs after CRC resection was suggested as independent prognostic marker of recurrence (Peach et al., 2010). It was concluded that the presence of CTCs in nonmetastatic colon cancer is rare and barely detectable with the only commercially available assay for determination of CTCs, the CellSearch system. Further studies are needed to clarify the optimal time point for blood sampling and the benefit of chemotherapy in CTC-positive patients with stage II disease. The low incidence of CTCs in nonmetastatic CRC requires highly sensitive and specific detection methods. A gastrointestinal-specific anti-CK20 antibody was developed by Wong et al. and demonstrated to detect CTCs in 58 of 101 patients with stage I-III CRC preoperatively and, furthermore, a decrease in CTCs in 51 of these 58 patients after surgery (Wong et al., 2009). Another study by this group found CK20 expression in lymph nodes and blood of CRC patients and a follow-up study reported that these cells predicted metastasis (Wong et al., 2009).

Recently, it was observed that CTCs are often undetected in metastatic breast cancer patients treated with bevacizumab (Gazzaniga et al., 2011). Due to the frequent use of bevacizumab as first-line medication for metastatic CRC, the predictive value of the CTC count in patients treated with first-line chemotherapy plus bevacizumab compared with those treated with chemotherapy plus cetuximab was investigated. In the bevacizumab-treated patient group the median number of baseline CTCs was 2.7/7.5 ml blood and dropped to zero in most patients. However, half of the apparently CTC-negative patients proved to have progressive disease. Thus, bevacizumab-induced hypoxia in the primary tumor may generate a selected population of cells undergoing epithelial-mesenchymal transformation (EMT) with downregulation of epithelial markers such as EpCAM and CKs making these cells undetectable by the CellSearch system. Mego et al. for the first time used the term 'undetectable CTCs' due to the obvious underestimation of CTCs that underwent EMT by the CellSearch system (Mego et al., 2011).

2.3 Surgery and tumor cell dissemination

Disturbing tumors mechanically, which may lead to shedding of cancer cells during surgery, constitutes a possible mechanism of tumor dissemination. The quantification of CTCs can be applied to assess the extent of this phenomenon. Lu et al. published a large-scale study involving stage III and IV CRC patients who underwent curative resections. This study found that postoperative relapse was strongly correlated with laparotomy versus laparoscopic surgery, lymph node metastases, as well as CTC levels if elevated at both pre- and postoperative time points (Lu et al., 2011). In contrast, another study reported no statistically significant difference of the $CD45^-/CK^+$ tumor cell count in the blood at time of surgical incision, after tumor resection and at the end of operation (Tralhão et al., 2010). A similar result was published by Wind et al. for the respective type of operative procedures, revealing that the cumulative percentage of samples containing CTCs was significantly higher during open surgery as compared to the laparoscopic approach (Wind et al., 2009). However, dissemination of CK^+ cells during surgery of hepatic metastases, a frequent event in colon cancer patients, did not predict extrahepatic recurrence (Schoppmeyer et al., 2006, Koch et al., 2007). In conclusion, CTCs seem to be generated during surgery; however, their significance for the occurrence of relapses is not clear.

2.4 Epithelial-mesenchymal transition (EMT) and CKs

EMT is considered an essential process in the metastatic cascade enabling the cells to aquire a mesenchymal cell phenotype characterized by increased motility and altered morphology

(Kalluri and Weinberg, 2009). The appearance of dot-like α-smooth muscle actin (α-SMA)-staining in CK^+ cells during tumor progression may indicate the initial phase of EMT in CRC (Valc et al., 2011). Increasing intraepithelial α-SMA concomitant with decreasing E-cadherin expression points to a loss of epithelial cell contact in the beginning of EMT. However, downregulation of epithelial markers like EpCAM and CKs in EMT-transformed tumor cells implicates the infeasibility to detect the most aggressive CTCs by methods relying on these markers (Mego et al., 2011). Epithelial cancer cells are likely to undergo EMT before they enter the peripheral circulation. Both EpCAM and CKs are downregulated as part of an oncogenic pathway promoting increased invasiveness and metastatic potential (Woelfle et al., 2004; Willipinski-Stapelfeldt et al., 2005). EpCAM is expressed in most but not all tumors and there is evidence for its modulation with cancer progression and metastasis (Mikolajczyk et al., 2011). Again, EpCAM expression may be suppressed to allow dissociation of epithelial cancer cells from the tumor and structural cytoplasmic CKs are downregulated to facilitate cell plasticity and migration. It is not always clear whether the loss of CKs is a result of independent oncogenic processes or whether it is always related to EMT. Aberrant occurrence of CKs in BM appears to be more common than in peripheral blood, and CK expression caused by inflammation can also contribute to false-positive observations (Dandachi et al., 2005). Although reduced expression of CK8 and CK20 is associated with EMT in CRC, which is generally indicative of higher tumor aggressiveness and decreased patient survival, several studies provided evidence supporting an active role of CKs in cancer cell invasion and metastasis (Knosel et al., 2006). Transfection of CK8 and CK18 into vimentin-positive mouse L fibroblasts resulted in higher migratory and invasive ability, indicating that CKs may influence cell shape and migration through interaction with the extracellular environment (Chu et al., 1993). Similarly, experimental coexpression of vimentin with CK8 and CK18 increases invasion and migration of human melanoma and breast cancer cells in vitro (Hendrix et al., 1997)

EMT in breast tumor cells is characterized by upregulation of expression of vimentin, Twist, Snail, Slug and Sip1, among others (Kalluri and Weinberg, 2009). A recent study in early and metastatic breast cancer patients found that immunomagnetic separation of CTCs and triple-immunofluorescence obtained with anti-CK/anti-Twist/anti-vimentin antibodies indicated that the mesenchymal marker could be coexpressed in the same CK^+ cell, since 64% of the total identified CTCs were triple-stained (Kallergi et al., 2011). Among patients with early disease, approximately half of the CK^+ CTCs were double-stained with anti-vimentin and anti-Twist antibodies, while the corresponding values for metastatic patients were 74% and 97%, respectively. The median expression of CK^+ $vimentin^+$ and CK^+ $Twist^+$ cells per patient in metastatic patients was nearly 100% and in an adjuvant chemotherapy setting approximately 50%, respectively. The high incidence of coexpressing cells in metastatic breast patients compared to early stage tumors point to a high metastatic potential of CTCs with EMT phenotype. Similar results were found for non-small cell lung cancer (NSCLC) and prostate tumor patients, where hybrid CTCs with an EMT phenotype coexpressing vimentin and CKs were detected (Lecharpentier et al., 2011; Armstrong et al., 2011). Furthermore, DTCs in BM may reverse EMT in a process termed mesenchymal-epithelial transition (MET) and regain an epithelial phenotype with loss of mesenchymal migratory properties (van der Pluijm, 2011). Therefore, antibodies to CKs are still expected to help in the identification of tumor cells that underwent EMT, dependent on the respective histological origin.

2.5 CK-positive CTCs and cancer stem cells (CSCs)

The CSC concept hypothesizes that tumors arise from a small population of stem cells, which may disseminate from the primary tumor to a stem cell niche until relapse. The relationship of cancer stem cells (CSCs) with CTCs is entirely unclear at this point. Thus, CTCs have additional intravasation and extravasation properties and, possibly, stem cell characteristics. CD133 (prominin) is one of the key markers of CSCs in CRC and CD133-positive cells have high tumorigenic ability in nude mice (Smirnov et al., 2005). Furthermore, it was reported that CSCs are often characterized by downregulation of epithelial markers such EpCAM and CKs. Stem cell markers are frequently overexpressed in CTCs of patients with metastatic breast cancer. This stem cell-like subpopulation of CTCs is characterized by a nonproliferative and chemoresistant phenotype (Lianidou & Markou, 2011). These facts would suggest that a new marker is necessary for the detection of CK-downregulated, aggressive CTCs, which may comprise CSCs as well. The surface markers of colon CSCs, namely CD133, CD44, CD166, Musashi-1, CD29, CD24, leucine-rich repeat-containing G-protein-coupled receptor 5 and aldehyde dehydrogenase 1 were reported (Dhawan et al., 2011). The clinical significance of CSC-like CTCs as a prognostic factor for OS and DFS in the peripheral blood of CRC patients was published (Iinuma, et al., 2011). CTCs of CRC patients who had undergone curative surgery expressed CEA, CK19, CK20 and/or CD133 mRNA in peripheral blood. In particular, these $CEA^{+}/CK^{+}/CD133^{+}$ CTCs demonstrated significant prognostic value in patients with Dukes' stage B and C cancer, but not Duke's A. Again, this finding demonstrates that CTCs with CSC characteristics can still express CKs and may be detected with respective pan-CK antibodies.

2.6 Soluble CK18 fragments as markers of residual tumor load

There are several reports dealing with determinations of CK fragments in BM samples of cancer patients. An investigation using BM aspirates of breast cancer patients reported a positive relationship between the detection of micrometastic tumor cells in immunocytochemistry with the pan-CK antibody A45-B/B3 and measurements of CK fragment CYFRA 21-1 expression (Pierga et al., 2004). CYFRA 21-1 was significantly elevated in patients with disseminated tumors and both markers were associated with a poorer survival for patients with stage I to III breast cancer. The CK-positive cells in BM aspirates were reported to lack expression of urokinase plasminogen activator which is associated with metastasis (Werther et al., 2002). In order to avoid tedious immunohistochemical methods, a new enzyme immunoassay for detection of occult tumor cells in BM was developed that was designed to detect intracellular CK19 released from epithelial tumor cells after they had been lysed by freezing/thawing cycles (Riethmüller et al., 1997). Comparison of immunohistochemistry with this new assays revealed higher incidence of epithelial cells in advanced T-stage of CRC patients by the ELISA test. In comparison with controls, BM samples of cancer patients were found to have significantly elevated levels of CK19 and in the analysis of almost 400 BM aspirates of cancer patients, a significant correlation of ELISA and immunohistochemistry to detect CK^{+} cells was observed. However, most discordant samples were ELISA-positive and the CK status detected by this method did not correlate with the TNM stage and the histological grading. This immunoassay was reported to allow for sensitive and specific detection of DTCs in a faster, less laborious and more objective manner compared to immunohistochemistry.

Quantification of soluble CK fragments that are shed by epithelial tumor cells by newer methods may serve as an alternative way for detection of occult residual tumor load by DTC counting. In particular, CK18, an intracellular, mainly insoluble protein highly expressed by various types of epithelial cells, is released in form of a caspase-cleaved 30 kD (ccCK18) and a 65 kD fragment into the extracellular compartment during apoptosis and necrosis, respectively, though active export of intact CK19 has also been reported (Linder, 2011; Alix-Panabieres et al, 2009). The 30 and 65 kD fragments can be quantified by the M30-Apoptosense® ELISA and the M65® ELISA assay (Peviva, Bromma, Sweden), respectively. So far, a single study has been conducted in small cell lung cancer (SCLC) patients undergoing standard chemotherapy to evaluate cell death assays detecting CK18 fragments (ccCK18 and M65) and CTC profiles using the CellSearch system (Hou et al., 2009). In this study both ccCK18 and M65 correlated with known clinical and biochemical prognostic factors including tumor stage and expression of lactate dehydrogenase. The number of CTCs had prognostic significance and correlated with pretreatment M65 levels. The accordance between levels of the circulating apoptotic-specific protein ccCK18 and the proportion of morphologically apoptotic CTCs corroborate the role of ccCK18 to indicate tumor cell apoptosis.

Although the levels of CKs in serum of cancer patients have been widely used for monitoring progression of tumor growth and effectiveness of treatment, the mechanisms of the release of CK fragments from cells is not clear (Linder et al., 2010). Studies in patients have shown that the release of CKs by tumors is a complex process, which seems to be not simply correlated to the number of proliferating cells or to the tumor mass but may also be dependent on the rate of cell damage (Oehr et al., 1997). During the development of CK18 as tumor marker the focus has switched from the perspective as proliferation marker to its significance as parameter of tumor cell death (Ausch et al., 2010). The demonstration of elevated levels of both ccCK18 and M65 in venous blood from tumors of endometrial cancer patients proved that these proteins were derived from the malignant tissue (Kramer et al., 2004). Additionally, and in contrast to the assumption that CKs are only released in fragmented form by epithelial cells as a result of necrosis/apoptosis, evidence for the active release of full-length CK19 by viable epithelial tumor cells was published (Alix-Panabieres et al., 2009). According to this study CK19-releasing cells were detected in BM of 44-70% of breast cancer patients and correlated to the presence of manifest metastases.

2.6.1 Effect of radical tumor surgery on circulating CK18 fragments in CRC patients

We quantified the CK18 fragments M65 and ccCK18 in serum samples of CRC patients pre- and postoperatively using ELISA assays and demonstrated higher levels of circulating M65 and ccCK18 in patients with either low grade tumors or disseminated metastatic CRCs in comparison to nontumor control individuals. Due to tumor surgery approximately 60% of the CRC patients responded with a mean drop of soluble M65 blood levels of 30%, while the remaining 40% of patients showed a mean increase of 40%, respectively (Ausch et al., 2009a). The group with increased postoperative levels of M65 was characterized by a higher incidence of BM-DTCs in comparison to patients with postoperatively normalizing M65. In the case of circulating ccCK18 almost 80% of patients exhibited a significant decrease of approximately 75% in response to tumor removal; however, the remaining 20% revealed a mean increase of 40% of these CK fragment levels postoperatively (Ausch, et al., 2009b). The frequency of BM-DTCs, as detected before surgery with help of the pan-CK antibody A45-B/B3, was not significantly different for these two groups of patients with normalizing and increased ccCK18 levels. However, the course of ccCK18 correlated well with an increased number of recurrences in the group with persisting serum fragment levels within a follow-up of three years (hazard ratio: 8.3). In conclusion, radical removal of the tumor, which is supposed to be the main source of the circulating CK18 fragments, failed to result in a decline of M65 levels to normal values in this subgroup of patients characterized by occurrence of BM-DTCs and increased risk of early relapses. In the same group of CRC patients the overall rate of BM-DTCs detected was 23% independent of the respective tumor stage. No difference was found in relapse and OS between patients with or without BM-DTCs preoperatively after a median follow-up of 35.4 months (Buxhofer-Ausch et al., 2009). The BM-DTC status was found to be changed for a second BM aspiration after twelve months in a quarter of the patients. Thus, failure to yield postoperative reduction of circulating CK18 fragments in individual CRC patients seems to be indicative of remaining tumor tissue.

CTCs released during surgery may undergo apoptotic cell death due to a failure of homing of the majority of cells to a suitable environment, while a minor fraction eventually manages to settle at distant sites and causes tumor recurrence (Rossi et al., 2010). Retsky et al. suggested that surgery to remove the primary tumor often terminates the dormancy DTCs resulting in accelerated relapses, as demonstrated in over half of the metastatic cases (Retsky et al., 2008). Another explanation for the CK release may be intracellular degradation of CK18 by caspases and shedding into the circulation as part of EMT without cell death or, alternatively, secretion of CK18 in intact form, as exemplified for CK19, followed by cleavage by caspases in the BM or serum (Alix-Panabieres et al, 2009).

2.6.2 Course of M65 concentrations in BM aspirates of CRC patients

In the present study we extended the measurement of M65 to BM aspirates of CRC patients obtained preoperatively and one year after surgery using the methods described by Ausch et al. (Ausch et al., 2009a).

2.6.2.1 Patients and methods

A total of 56 patients with colorectal cancer who were treated between January 2002 and December 2004 at the Donauspital, Vienna and had a follow-up period of more than 3 years. 30 patients underwent surgery for primary colorectal carcinoma and none of the patients had received chemotherapy and/or radiotherapy prior to surgery. All patients were checked for infections by viral tests, blood count and chemistry, including determination of C-reactive protein. Twenty-three nontumor patients admitted to the outpatient department for minor complaints served as controls. Collected blood was centrifuged 2000 rpm for 10 minutes and stored at -20 °C. Written informed consent was obtained from all patients. The study was approved by the local ethics committee and the institutional review board. BM aspirates were obtained from both upper iliac crests (5ml each) by needle aspiration immediately prior to the operation under general anesthesia. Mononuclear cells of bone marrow aspirates were separated by Ficoll-Hypaque density gradient centrifugation (GE Healthcare, Little Chalfont, UK). Cytospins containing $1x10^6$ cells/slide were fixed in acetone and stained using pancytokeratin pan-CK antibody A45-B/B3 (Micromet, Munich,

Germany; final concentration 5 µg/ml; 20 min). All staining steps, including blocking and washes, were performed using the Idetect-Super- Stain-(alkaline phosphatase)-Fast-Red kit according to the manufacturer's instruction (ID Labs, London, ON, Canada) and mouse monoclonal isotype controls were included. For assessment of BM-DTCs at least $2x10^6$ cells per specimen were screened blinded by two pathologists and a minimum of one tumor cell per $2x10^6$ mononuclear cells was regarded as a positive result for A45-B/B3. From all BM aspirates the concentrations of ccCK18 and and total CK18 (M65) were determined using the M30-Apoptosense® and the M65-ELISA assay® according to the manufacturer's instruction (Peviva, Bromma, Sweden), respectively. The coefficient of variance for the duplicate measurements of M30/M65 was < 7.5%.

2.6.2.2 Result of determinations of M65 in BM aspirates of CRC patients

The comparison of M65 concentrations determined from 30 CRC patients is shown in Figure 1. In the group of 16 patients with significant reduction (>10 %) of BM M65 levels, four cases of local relapses (Pat. # 2, 14, 52 and 68) were observed, whereas all four systemic relapses (Pat. # 3, 11, 43 and 45) occured in the second group who exhibited increasing M65 levels or minor reduction of <10%. Thus, the difference in respect to systemic relapses was highly significant (0/16 versus 4/14; 0 versus 28.6%; $p < 0.001$; Fisher's exact test). Mean differences of M65 for the two groups and the two time points were -42.5 ± 17.2% and +12.3 ± 19.2%, respectively. Obviously, the determination of BM M65 levels is not adequate to predict local relapses in CRC patients, but systemic relapses in this small group of CRC patients correlated with perioperative changes in this CK fragment. The course of BM M65 levels during the first postoperative year was studied for the BM DTC-positive and -negative groups. Assessment of the BM for pan-CK-positive tumor cells by inspection of two million mononuclear cells showed no correlation with the course of M65 for the first year after surgery: M65 decreased by -24.0 ± 36.8% for the BM-DTC-positive (n = 15) and by -9.8 ± 28.0% for the BM-DTC-negative patient group (n = 15), respectively. The former group comprised two systemic relapses while the latter exhibited two systemic and one local relapses (difference not significant). Although BM-DTCs were detected in 50% of these CRC patients, the status of BM did not correlate with the frequency of relapses during the follow-up of five years. However, analysis of BM-DTCs was performed without any enrichment of tumor cells and the analysis of CTCs actually seems to be more suitable to obtain prognostic results (Allen & El-Deiry, 2010). In most cases, concentrations of M65 in BM and peripheral blood showed good correlation (Olszewski-Hamilton et al., 2011). In conclusion, a reduction of BM M65 concentrations during the first postoperative year points to PFS in respect to systemic disease, whereas an increase or a minor reduction seems to be associated with residual tumor load and systemic recurrence. Increased preoperative or pretreatment blood concentration of M65 was described as independent prognostic parameter, possible reflecting tumor burden of the individual patients. However, the individual time courses of CK fragments may more accurate mirror the effects of tumor treatment. Although determination of the individual differences in circulating CK18 levels before and after tumor surgery is prone to interference by inflammation and benign disease, it represents a cost-effective alternative to the expensive automated counting of CTCs in nonmetastatic CRC. However, these results were obtained in a small group of CRC patients and need to be confirmed in a larger study.

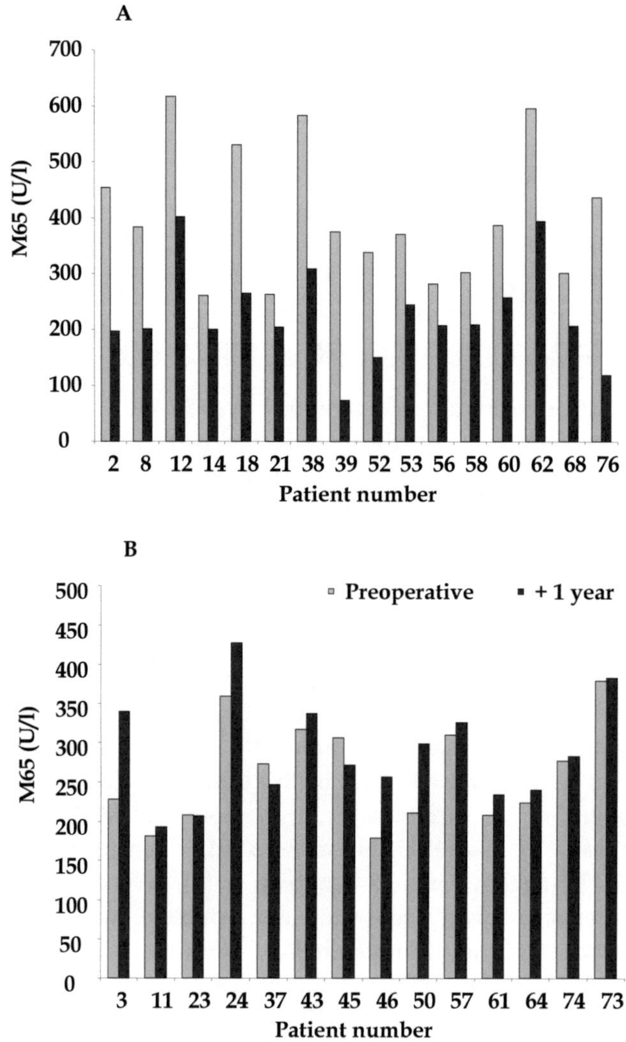

Fig. 1. Comparison of the differences of BM M65 concentrations in two CRC patient groups between preoperative and follow-up samples taken one year later. 30 patients were classified into a group of 16 showing significant reduction (>10%) of the BM M65 concentrations during the first year after surgery (A) and a group of 14 patients exhibiting <10% reduction of M65 (B). Data are shown as mean values (SD <10%).

3. Conclusions

Dissemination of tumor cells from primary tumors in the circulation seems to be an early event in tumor development for specific histological types. The presence of these DTCs in peripheral blood, bone marrow and distant organs is tested for providing the rationale for adjuvant systemic treatment (Bidard et al., 2011; Lin et al., 2011). Detection of DTC in bone marrow aspirates from breast cancer patients and other solid tumors at the primary diagnosis impacts the prognosis of disease. Technological advances in immunological and quantitative real-time PCR-based analysis allow for detection, enumeration and characterization of disseminated tumor cells in cancer patients. Proof of the expression of CKs by use of antibodies is the mainstay of most methods to detect DTCs and gain prognostic data of patients with carcinomas. Despite assumed downregulation of epithelial markers like CKs, during EMT they are still expressed in vimentin-positive hybrid CTCs and allow for the assessment of tumor dissemination. Determinations of individual courses of the levels of circulating CK fragments before and after tumor surgery in blood or BM of CRC patients seem to constitute a valuable technique to prove residual tumor load, provided that these CK fragments are not released due to nontumor causes. The advantage of measuring CK fragments in the circulation or BM aspirates may be the sensitive detection of DTCs independent of their localization. For reliable results in regard to systemic relapses careful monitoring of individual time courses of the levels of the CK fragments in tumor patients seem to be necessary.

4. Acknowledgment

This work was supported in part by a grant project no. 09003 from the "Bürgermeisterfond der Stadt Wien.

5. References

Allard, WJ., Matera, J., Miller, MC. Repollet, M., Connelly, MC., Rao, C., Tibbe, AG., Uhr, JW. & Terstappen, LW. (2004) Tumor cells circulate in the peripheral blood of all major carcinomas but not in healthy subjects or patients with nonmalignant diseases. *Clin Cancer Res* Vol. 10, no. 20, pp. 6897–6904

Alix-Panabieres, C., Vendrell, J.P., Slijper, M., Pelle, O., Barbotte, E., Mercier, G., Jacot,W., Fabbro, M. & Pantel, K. (2009) Full length cytokeratin-19 is released by human tumor cells: a potential role in metastatic progression of breast cancer. *Breast Cancer Res* Vol. 11, R39

Allen, J.E. & El-Deiry, W.S. (2010) Circulating Tumor Cells and Colorectal Cancer. *Curr Colorectal Cancer Rep* Vol. 6, no. 4, pp. 212-220

Allen-Mersh, TG., McCullough, TK., Patel, H., Wharton, RQ., Glover, C. & Jonas, SK. (2007) Role of circulating tumour cells in predicting recurrence after excision of primary colorectal carcinoma. *Br J Surg* Vol. 94, no. 1, pp. 96–105

Armstrong, A.J., Marengo, M.S., Oltean, S., Kemeny, G., Bitting, R.L., Turnbull, J.D., Herold, C.I., Marcom, P.K., George, D.J. & Garcia-Blanco, M.A. (2011) Circulating tumor cells from patients with advanced prostate and breast cancer display both epithelial and mesenchymal markers. *Mol Cancer Res* Vol. 9, no. 8, pp. 997-1007

Ausch, C., Buxhofer-Ausch, V., Olszewski, U., Schiessel, R., Ogris, E., Hinterberger, W. & Hamilton, G. (2009a) Circulating cytokeratin 18 fragment M65-a potential marker of malignancy in colorectal cancer patients. *J Gastrointest Surg* Vol. 13, no. 11, pp. 2020-2026

Ausch, C., Buxhofer-Ausch, V., Olszewski, U., Hinterberger, W., Ogris, E., Schiessel, R. & Hamilton, G. (2009b) Caspase-cleaved cytokeratin 18 fragment (M30) as marker of postoperative residual tumor load in colon cancer patients. *Eur J Surg Oncol* Vol. 35, pp. 1164–1168

Ausch, C., Buxhofer-Ausch, V., Olszewski, U. & Hamilton, G. (2010) Circulating cytokeratin 18 fragments and activation of dormant tumor cells in bone marrow of cancer patients. *Exp Therap Med* Vol. 1, pp. 9-12

Barak, CV., Goike, H., Panaretakism, KW. & Einarsson, R. (2004) Clinical utility of cytokeratins as tumor markers. *Clinical Biochemistry* Vol. 37, pp. 529-540

Bidard, FC., Ferrand, FR., Huguet, F., Hammel, P., Louvet, C., Malka, D., Boige, V., Ducreux, M., Andre, T., de Gramont, A., Mariani, P. & Pierga, JY. (2011) Disseminated and circulating tumor cells in gastrointestinal oncology. *Crit Rev Oncol* Hematol 2011, in press.

Bragulla, HH. & Homberger, DG. (2009) Structure and functions of keratin proteins in simple., stratified., keratinized and cornified epithelia. *J Anat* Vol. 214, pp. 516–559

Braun, S., Pantel, K., Müller, P., Janni, W., Hepp, F., Kentenich, CR., Gastroph, S., Wischnik, A., Dimpfl, T., Kindermann, G., Riethmüller, G. & Schlimok G. (2000) Cytokeratin-positive cells in the bone marrow and survival of patients with stage I, II, or III breast cancer. *N Engl J Med* Vol. 342, no. 8, pp. 525-533

Buxhofer-Ausch, V., Ausch, C., Kitzweger, E., Mollik, M., Reiner-Concin, A., Ogris, E., Stampfl, M., Hamilton, G., Schiessel, R. & Hinterberger, W. (2010) Spontaneous changes in tumour cell dissemination to bone marrow in colorectal cancer. *Colorectal Dis* Vol. 12, no. 8, pp. 776-782

Catenacci, DV., Kozloff, M., Kindler, HL, & Polite, B. (2011) Personalized colon cancer care in 2010. *Semin Oncol* Vol. 38, no. 2, pp. 284-308

Chu, YW., Runyan, RB., Oshima, RG. & Hendrix, MJ. (1993) Expression of complete keratin filaments in mouse L cells augments cell migration and invasion. *Proc Natl Acad Sci USA* Vol. 90, pp. 4261–4265

Cohen, SJ., Alpaugh, RK., Gross, S., O'Hara, SM., Smirnov, DA., Terstappen, LW., Allard, WJ., Bilbee, M., Cheng, JD., Hoffman, JP., Lewis, NL., Pellegrino, A., Rogatko, A., Sigurdson, E., Wang, H., Watson, JC., Weiner, LM. & Meropol NJ. (2006) Isolation and characterization of circulating tumor cells in patients with metastatic colorectal cancer. *Clin Colorectal Cancer* Vol. 6, no. 2, pp. 125-132

Cohen, SJ., Punt, C.J., Iannotti, N., Saidman, B.H., Sabbath, K.D., Gabrail, N.Y., Picus, J., Morse, M.A., Mitchell, E., Miller, MC., Doyle, G.V., Tissing H., Terstappen, L.W.& Meropol, N.J. (2009) Prognostic significance of circulating tumor cells in patients with metastatic colorectal cancer. *Ann Oncol* Vol. 20, no. 7, pp. 1223-1229

Coulombe, PA., Hutton, ME., Letai, A., Hebert, A., Paller, AS. & Fuchs, E. (1991) Point mutations in human keratin 14 genes of epidermolysis bullosa simplex patients, genetic and functional analyses. *Cell* Vol. 66, pp. 1301–1311

Cristofanilli M, Broglio KR, Guarneri V, et al. Circulating tumor cells in metastatic breast cancer: biologic staging beyond tumor burden. *Clin Breast Cancer* Vol. 7, no. 6, pp. 471–479

Dandachi, N., Balic, M., Stanzer, S., Halm, M., Resel, M., Hinterleitner, TA., Samonigg, H. & Bauernhofer T. (2005) Critical evaluation of real-time reverse transcriptase-polymerase chain reaction for the quantitative detection of cytokeratin 20 mRNA in colorectal cancer patients. *J Mol Diagn* Vol. 7, no. 5, pp. 631-637

Dhawan, P., Ahmad, R., Srivastava, AS. & Singh, AB. (2011) Cancer stem cells and colorectal cancer: an overview. *Curr Top Med Chem* Vol. 11, no. 3, pp. 1592-1598

Flatmark, K., Borgen, E., Nesland, J.M., Rasmussen, H., Johannessen, HO., Bukholm, I., Rosales, R., Hårklau, L., Jacobsen, HJ., Sandstad, B., Boye, K. & Fodstad, Ø. (2011) Disseminated tumour cells as a prognostic biomarker in colorectal cancer. *Br J Cancer* Vol. 104, no. 9, pp. 1434-1439

Gangadhar, T., Schilsky, RL. & Medscape. (2010) Molecular markers to individualize adjuvant therapy for colon cancer. *Nat Rev Clin Oncol* Vol. 7, no. 6, pp. 318-325

Gazzaniga, P., Raimondi, C., Gradilone, A., Di Seri, M., Longo, F., Cortesi, E. & Frati L. (2011) Circulating tumor cells, colon cancer and bevacizumab: the meaning of zero. *Ann Oncol* Vol. 22, no. 8, pp. 1929-1930

Harrison, S. & Benziger, H. (2011) The molecular biology of colorectal carcinoma and its implications: a review. *Surgeon* Vol. 9, no. 4, pp. 200-210

Hendrix, MJ., Seftor, EA., Seftor, RE. & Trevor, KT. (1997) Experimental co-expression of vimentin and keratin intermediate filaments in human breast cancer cells results in phenotypic interconversion and increased invasive behavior. *Am J Pathol* Vol. 150, pp. 483–495

Hou, JM., Greystoke, A., Lancashire, L., Cummings, J., Ward. T., Board, R., Amir, E., Hughes, S., Krebs, M., Hughes, A., Ranson, M., Lorigan, P., Dive, C. & Blackhall, FH. (2009) Evaluation of circulating tumor cells and serological cell death biomarkers in small cell lung cancer patients undergoing chemotherapy. *Am J Pathol* Vol. 175, no. 2, pp. 808-816

Iddings, D & Bilchik, A. (2007) The biologic significance of micrometastatic disease and sentinel lymph node technology on colorectal cancer. *J Surg Oncol* Vol. 96, pp. 671-677

Iinuma, H., Watanabe, T., Mimori, K., Adachi, M., Hayashi, N., Tamura, J., Matsuda K., Fukushima, R., Okinaga, K., Sasako, M. & Mori, M. (2011) Clinical significance of circulating tumor cells, including cancer stem-like cells, in peripheral blood for recurrence and prognosis in patients with Dukes' stage B and C colorectal cancer. *J Clin Oncol* Vol. 29, no. 12, pp. 1547-1555

Jaitovich, A., Mehta, S., Na, N., Ciechanover, A., Goldman, R.D. & Ridge, K.M. (2008) Ubiquitin-proteasome-mediated degradation of keratin intermediate filaments in mechanically stimulated A549 cells. *J Biol Chem* 283, no. 37, pp. 25348–25355

Kallergi, G., Papadaki, M.A., Politaki, E., Mavroudis, D., Georgoulias, V. & Agelaki, S. (2011) Epithelial to mesenchymal transition markers expressed in circulating tumour cells of early and metastatic breast cancer patients. *Breast Cancer Res* Vol. 13, no. 3, R59

Kalluri, R. & Weinberg, RA. (2009) The basics of epithelial-mesenchymal transition. *J Clin Invest* Vol. 119, no. 6, pp. 1420-1428

Karantza, V. (2011) Keratins in health and cancer, more than mere epithelial cell markers. *Oncogene* Vol. 30, no. 2, pp. 127-138

Kim, MY., Oskarsson, T., Acharyya, S., Nguyen, DX., Zhang, XH., Norton, L. & Massagué, J. (2009) Tumor self-seeding by circulating cancer cells. *Cell* Vol. 139, no. 7, pp. 1315-1326

Knosel, T., Emde, V., Schluns, K., Schlag, PM., Dietel, M. & Petersen, I. (2006) Cytokeratin profiles identify diagnostic signatures in colorectal cancer using multiplex analysis of tissue microarrays. *Cell Oncol* Vol. 28, pp. 167–175

Koch, M., Kienle, P., Kastrati, D., Antolovic, D., Schmidt, J., Herfarth, C., von Knebel Doeberitz, M. & Weitz, J. (2006) Prognostic impact of hematogenous tumor cell dissemination in patients with stage II colorectal cancer. *Int J Cancer* Vol. 118, no. 12, pp. 3072–3077

Koch, M., Kienle, P., Logan, E., Antolovic, D., Galindo, L., Schmitz-Winnenthal, FH., Schmidt, J., Herfarth, C. & Weitz, J. (2007) Detection of disseminated tumor cells in liver biopsies of colorectal cancer patients is not associated with a worse prognosis. *Ann Surg Oncol* Vol. 14, no. 2, pp. 810-817

Kongara, S., Kravchuk, O., Teplova, I., Lozy, F., Schulte, J., Moore, D., Barnard, N., Neumann, CA., White, E. & Karantza, V. (2010) Autophagy regulates keratin 8 homeostasis in mammary epithelial cells and in breast tumors. *Mol Cancer Res* Vol. 8, pp. 873–884

Kramer, G., Erdal, H., Mertens, HJ., Nap, M., Mauermann, J., Steiner, G., Marberger, M., Bivén, K., Shoshan, MC. & Linder, S. (2004) Differentiation between cell death modes using measurements of different soluble forms of extracellular cytokeratin 18. *Cancer Res* Vol. 64, no. 5, pp. 1751-1756

Ku, NO., Liao, J. & Omary, MB. (1997) Apoptosis generates stable fragments of human type I keratins. *J Biol Chem* Vol. 272, no. 52, pp. 33197-33203

Lin, H., Balic, M., Zheng, S., Datar, R. & Cote, RJ. (2011). Disseminated and circulating tumor cells: Role in effective cancer management. *Crit Rev Oncol Hematol* Vol. 77, no. 1, pp. 1-11

Linder, S. (2007) Cytokeratin Markers Come of Age. Tumor Biol Vol. 28, pp. 189-195

Linder, S., Olofsson, MH., Herrmann, R. & Ulukaya, E. (2010) Utilization of cytokeratin-based biomarkers for pharmacodynamic studies. *Expert Rev Mol Diagn* Vol. 10, pp. 353–359

Linder, S. (2011) Caspase-cleaved keratin 18 as a biomarker for non-alcoholic steatohepatitis (NASH) - The need for correct terminology. *J Hepatol* Vol. 55, no. 6, p. 1467.

Lecharpentier, A., Vielh, P., Perez-Moreno, P., Planchard, D., Soria, J.C. & Farace, F. (2011) Detection of circulating tumour cells with a hybrid (epithelial/mesenchymal) phenotype in patients with metastatic non-small cell lung cancer. *Br J Cancer* 2011, in press.

Lianidou, ES. & Markou, A. (2011) Circulating tumor cells in breast cancer: detection systems, molecular characterization, and future challenges. *Clin Chem* Vol. 57, no. 9, pp. 1242-1255

Lu, CY., Uen, YH., Tsai, HL., Chuang, SC., Hou, MF., Wu, DC., Hank Juo, SH., Lin, SR. & Wang, JY. (2011) Molecular detection of persistent postoperative circulating tumour cells in stages II and III colon cancer patients via multiple blood sampling: prognostic significance of detection for early relapse. *Br J Cancer* Vol. 104, no. 7, pp. 1178-1184

Lugo, TG., Braun, S., Cote, RJ., Pantel, K. & Rusch, V. (2003) Detection and measurement of occult disease for the prognosis of solid tumors. *J Clin Oncol* Vol. 21, no. 13, pp. 2609–2615

Luzzi, KJ., MacDonald, IC., Schmidt, EE., Kerkvliet, N., Morris, VL., Chambers, AF. & Groom, AC. (1998) Multistep nature of metastatic inefficiency: dormancy of solitary cells after successful extravasation and limited survival of early micrometastases. *Am J Pathol* Vol. 153, no. 3, pp. 865-873

Maestro, LM., Sastre, J., Rafael, SB., Veganzones, SB., Vidaurreta, M., Martín, M., Olivier, C., De La Orden, VB., Garcia-Saenz, JA., Alfonso, R., Arroyo, M. & Diaz-Rubio, E.

(2009) Circulating tumor cells in solid tumor in metastatic and localized stages. *Anticancer Res* Vol. 29, no. 11, pp. 4839-4843

Mani, SA., Guo, W., Liao, MJ., Eaton, EN., Ayyanan, A., Zhou, AY., Brooks, M., Reinhard, F., Zhang, CC., Shipitsin, M., Campbell, LL., Polyak, K., Brisken, C., Yang, J. & Weinberg, RA. (2008) The epithelial-mesenchymal transition generates cells with properties of stem cells. *Cell* Vol. 133, no. 4, pp. 704-715

Mego, M., Mani, SA., Lee, BN., Li, C., Evans, KW., Cohen, EN., Gao, H., Jackson, SA., Giordano, A., Hortobagyi, GN., Cristofanilli, M., Lucci, A. & Reuben, JM. Expression of epithelial-mesenchymal transition-inducing transcription factors in primary breast cancer: The effect of neoadjuvant therapy. *Int J Cancer* 2011, in press.

Mikolajczyk, SD., Millar, LS., Tsinberg, P., Coutts, SM., Zomorrodi, M., Pham, T., Bischoff, FZ. & Pircher, TJ. (2011) Detection of EpCAM-Negative and Cytokeratin-Negative Circulating Tumor Cells in Peripheral Blood. *J Oncol* 2011, 252361

Miller, MC., Doyle, GV. & Terstappen, LW. (2010) Significance of Circulating Tumor Cells Detected by the CellSearch System in Patients with Metastatic Breast Colorectal and Prostate Cancer. *J Oncol* 2010, 617421.

Moll, R., Franke, WW., Schiller, DL., Geiger, B. & Krepler, R. (1982) The catalog of human cytokeratins, patterns of expression in normal epithelia., tumors and cultured cells. *Cell* Vol. 31, no. 1, pp. 11–24

Mostert, B., Sleijfer, S., Foekens, JA. & Gratama, JW. (2009) Circulating tumor cells (CTCs): detection methods and their clinical relevance in breast cancer. *Cancer Treat Rev* Vol. 35, no. 5, pp. 463–474

Na, N., Chandel, NS., Litvan, J. & Ridge, KM. (2010) Mitochondrial reactive oxygen species are required for hypoxia-induced degradation of keratin intermediate filaments. *FASEB J* Vol. 24, no. 3, pp. 799–809

Nelson, DA., Tan, TT., Rabson, AB., Anderson, D., Degenhardt, K. & White, E. (2004) Hypoxia and defective apoptosis drive genomic instability and tumorigenesis. *Genes Dev* Vol. 18, pp. 2095–2107

Negin, BP. & Cohen, SJ. (2010) Circulating tumor cells in colorectal cancer: past, present, and future challenges. *Curr Treat Options Oncol* Vol. 11, no. 1-2, pp. 1-13

Novaes, M., Bendit, I., Garicochea B. & del Giglio, A. (1997) Reverse transcriptase-polymerase chain reaction analysis of cytokeratin 19 expression in the peripheral blood mononuclear cells of normal female blood donors. *Mol Pathol* Vol. 50, no. 4, pp. 209–211

O'Connell, JB.; Maggard, MA. & Ko, CY. (2004) Colon cancer survival rates with the new American Joint Committee on Cancer sixth edition staging. *J Natl Cancer Inst* Vol. 96, no. 19, 1420–1425

Oehr, P., Vacata, V., Ruhlmann, J. & Rink, H. (1997) Computer modeling of cytokeratin release in clinical oncology. *Anticancer Res* Vol. 17, no. 4B, pp. 3111-3112

Olszewski-Hamilton, U., Ausch, C., Buxhofer-Ausch, V. & Hamilton, G. (2011) Significance of Cytokeratin Fragment M65 and Cytokines IL6, IL8 and IL17A in Bone Marrow Aspirates of Colorectal Cancer Patients. *BJMMR* Vol. 1, no. 4, pp. 170-181

Omary, MB., Ku, NO., Strnad, P. & Hanada, S. (2009) Toward unraveling the complexity of simple epithelial keratins in human disease. *J Clin Invest* Vol. 119, pp. 1794–1805

Pantel, K., Schlimok, G., Angstwurm, M., Weckermann, D., Schmaus, W., Gath, H., Passlick B., Izbicki, JR. & Riethmuller G. (1994) Methodological analysis of immunocytochemical screening for disseminated epithelial tumor cells in bone marrow. *J Hematother* Vol. 3, pp. 165–173

Pantel, K., Brakenhoff, RH. & Brandt B. (2008) Detection, clinical relevance and specific biological properties of disseminating tumour cells. *Nature Rev Cancer* Vol. 8, no. 5, pp. 329–340

Pantel, K. & Alix-Panabières, C. (2010) Circulating tumour cells in cancer patients: challenges and perspectives. *Trends Mol Med* Vol. 16, no. 9, pp. 398-406

Paterlini-Brechot, P. & Benali, NL. (2007) Circulating tumor cells (CTC) detection: clinical impact and future directions. *Cancer Lett* Vol. 253, no. 2, pp. 180–204

Peach, G., Kim, C., Zacharakis, E., Purkayastha, S. & Ziprin, P. (2010) Prognostic significance of circulating tumor cells following surgical resection of colorectal cancers: a systematic review. *Br J Cancer* Vol. 102, no. 9, pp. 1327-1334

Pierga, JY., Deneux, L., Bonneton, C., Vincent-Salomon, A., Nos, C., Anract, P., Magdelénat, H., Pouillart, P. & Thiery, JP. (2004) Prognostic value of cytokeratin 19 fragment (CYFRA 21-1) and cytokeratin-positive cells in bone marrow samples of breast cancer patients. *Int J Biol Markers* Vol. 19, no.1, pp. 23-31

van der Pluijm, G. (2011) Epithelial plasticity, cancer stem cells and bone metastasis formation. *Bone* Vol. 48, No. 1, pp. 37-43.

Rahbari, NN., Aigner, M., Thorlund, K., Mollberg, N., Motschall, E., Jensen, K., Diener, MK., Büchler, MW., Koch, M. & Weitz, J. (2010) Meta-analysis shows that detection of circulating tumor cells indicates poor prognosis in patients with colorectal cancer. *Gastroenterology* Vol. 138, no. 5, pp. 1714-1726

Rao, CG., Chianese, D., Doyle, GV., Miller, MC., Russell, T., Sanders, RA. Jr & Terstappen LW. (2005) Expression of epithelial cell adhesion molecule in carcinoma cells present in blood and primary and metastatic tumors. *Int J Oncol* Vol. 27, no. 1, pp. 49–57

Retsky, MW., Demicheli, R., Hrushesky, WJ., Baum, M. & Gukas, ID. (2008) Dormancy and surgery-driven escape from dormancy help explain some clinical features of breast cancer. *APMIS* Vol. 116, pp. 730-741

Riethdorf, S., Wikman, H., Pantel, K. (2008) Review: Biological relevance of disseminated tumor cells in cancer patients. *Int J Cancer* Vol. 123, no. 9, pp. 1991-2006

Höchtlen-Vollmar, W., Gruber, R., Bodenmüller, H., Felber, E., Lindemann, F., Passlick, B., Schlimok, G., Pantel, K. & Riethmüller, G. (1997) Occult epithelial tumor cells detected in bone marrow by an enzyme immunoassay specific for cytokeratin 19. *Int J Cancer* Vol. 70, no. 4, pp. 396-400

Rossi, E., Basso, U., Celadin, R., Zilio, F., Pucciarelli, S., Aieta, M., Barile, C., Sava, T., Bonciarelli, G., Tumolo, S., Ghiotto, C., Magro, C., Jirillo, A., Indraccolo, S., Amadori, A.& Zamarchi R. (2010) M30 neoepitope expression in epithelial cancer: quantification of apoptosis in circulating tumor cells by CellSearch analysis. *Clin Cancer Res* Vol. 16, no. 21, pp. 5233-5243

Saijo, N. (2011) Critical comments for roles of biomarkers in the diagnosis and treatment of cancer. *Cancer Treat Rev* Vol. 38, no. 1, pp. 63-67

Sastre, J., Maestro, ML., Puente, J., Veganzones, S., Alfonso, R., Rafael, S., García-Saenz, JA., Vidaurreta, M., Martín, M., Arroyo, M., Sanz-Casla, MT. & Díaz-Rubio, E. (2008) Circulating tumor cells in colorectal cancer: correlation with clinical and pathological variables. *Ann Oncol* Vol. 19, no. 5, pp. 935-938

Sato, N.; Hayashi, N.; Imamura, Y.; Tanaka, Y.; Kinoshita, K.; Kurashige, J.; Saito, S.; Karashima, R.; Hirashima, K.; Nagai, Y.; Miyamoto, Y.; Iwatsuki, M.; Baba, Y.; Watanabe M. & Baba, H. (2011) Usefulness of Transcription-Reverse Transcription Concerted Reaction Method for Detecting Circulating Tumor Cells in Patients With Colorectal Cancer. *Ann Surg Oncol* 2011, in press.

Scott, LC., Evans, TR., Cassidy, J., Harden, S., Paul, J., Ullah, R., O'Brien, V. & Brown, R. (2009) Cytokeratin 18 in plasma of patients with gastrointestinal adenocarcinoma as a biomarker of tumour response. *Br J Cancer* Vol. 101, no. 4, pp. 410-417

Schoppmeyer, K., Frühauf, N., Oldhafer, K., Seeber, S. & Kasimir-Bauer, S. (2006) Tumor cell dissemination in colon cancer does not predict extrahepatic recurrence in patients undergoing surgery for hepatic metastases. *Oncol Rep* Vol. 15, no. 2, pp. 449-454

Sergeant, G.; Penninckx, F. & Topal, B. (2008) Quantitative RT-PCR detection of colorectal tumor cells in peripheral blood a systematic review. *J Surg Res* Vol. 150, no. 1, pp. 144-152

Smirnov, DA., Zweitzig, DR., Foulk, BW., Miller, MC., Doyle, GV., Pienta, KJ., Meropol, NJ., Weiner, LM., Cohen, SJ., Moreno, JG., Connelly, MC., Terstappen, LW. & O'Hara, SM. (2005) Global gene expression profiling of circulating tumor cells. *Cancer Res* Vol. 65, no. 12, pp. 4993-4997

Thorsteinsson, M., Söletormos, G. & Jess, P. (2011a) Low number of detectable circulating tumor cells in non-metastatic colon cancer. *Anticancer Res* Vol. 31, no. 2, pp. 613-617

Thorsteinsson, M. & Jess, P. (2011b) The clinical significance of circulating tumor cells in non-metastatic colorectal cancer--a review. *Eur J Surg Oncol* Vol. 37, no. 6, pp. 459-465

Tol, J., Koopman, M., Miller, MC., Tibbe, A., Cats, A., Creemers, GJ., Vos, AH., Nagtegaal, ID., Terstappen, LW. & Punt, CJ. (2010) Circulating tumour cells early predict progression-free and overall survival in advanced colorectal cancer patients treated with chemotherapy and targeted agents. *Ann Oncol* Vol. 21, no. 5, pp. 1006-1012

Tralhão, JG., Hoti, E., Serôdio, M., Laranjeiro, P., Paiva, A., Abrantes, AM., Pais, ML., Botelho, MF. & Castro Sousa, F. (2010) Perioperative tumor cell dissemination in patients with primary or metastatic colorectal cancer. *Eur J Surg Oncol* Vol. 36, no. 2, pp. 125-129

Van Schaeybroeck, S., Allen, WL., Turkington, RC. & Johnston, PG. (2011) Implementing prognostic and predictive biomarkers in CRC clinical trials. *Nat Rev Clin Oncol* Vol. 8, no. 4, pp. 222-232

Valcz, G., Sipos, F., Krenács, T., Molnár, J., Patai, A.V., Leiszter, K., Tóth, K., Wichmann, B., Molnár, B. & Tulassay, Z. (2011) Increase of α-SMA(+) and CK (+) Cells as an Early Sign of Epithelial-Mesenchymal Transition during Colorectal Carcinogenesis. *Pathol Oncol Res*. 2011, in press.

Werther K, Normark M, Brünner N, Nielsen HJ. (2002) Cytokeratin-positive cells in preoperative peripheral blood and bone marrow aspirates of patients with colorectal cancer. *Scand J Clin Lab Invest* Vol. 62, no. 1, pp. 49-57

Willipinski-Stapelfeldt, B., Riethdorf, S., Assmann, V., Woelfle, U., Rau, T., Sauter, G., Heukeshoven, J. & Pantel, K. (2005) Changes in cytoskeletal protein composition indicative of an epithelial-mesenchymal transition in human micrometastatic and primary breast carcinoma cells. *Clin Cancer Res* Vol. 11, no. 22, pp. 8006-8014

Wind, J., Tuynman, JB., Tibbe, AGJ, Swennenhuis, JF., Richel, DJ., van Berge Henegouwen, MI. & Bemelman, WA. (2009) Circulating tumour cells during laparoscopic and open surgery for primary colonic cancer in portal and peripheral blood. *Europ J Surg Oncol* Vol. 35, no. 9, pp. 942–950

Woelfle, U., Sauter, G., Santjer, S., Brakenhoff, R. & Pantel, K. (2004) Down-regulated expression of cytokeratin 18 promotes progression of human breast cancer. *Clin Cancer Res* Vol. 10, no. 8, pp. 2670–2674

Wong, SC., Chan, CM., Ma, BB., Hui, EP., Ng, SS., Lai, PB., Cheung, MT., Lo, ES., Chan, AK., Lam, MY., Au, TC. & Chan, AT. (2009) Clinical significance of cytokeratin 20-positive circulating tumor cells detected by a refined immunomagnetic enrichment assay in colorectal cancer patients. *Clin Cancer Res* Vol. 15, no. 3, pp. 1005–1012

7

FISH Probe Counting in Circulating Tumor Cells

Sjoerd T. Ligthart, Joost F. Swennenhuis,
Jan Greve and Leon W.M.M. Terstappen
University of Twente
The Netherlands

1. Introduction

Presence of tumor cells in blood of patients with metastatic carcinomas has been associated with poor progression free and overall survival (Cohen et al., 2008; Cristofanilli et al., 2004; de Bono et al., 2008). Assessment of treatment targets on circulating tumor cells (CTC) before initiation of therapy may provide a means to guide therapy (Attard et al., 2009; de Bono et al., 2007; Hayes et al., 2002; Meng et al., 2006; Meng et al., 2004; Smirnov et al., 2005; Swennenhuis et al., 2009). Characterization of CTC can be performed by Fluorescence In Situ Hybridization (FISH) which has been used to prove that CTC are indeed malignant (Fehm et al., 2002; Swennenhuis, et al., 2009), and that gene amplifications, deletions and translocations related to certain therapies can be detected (Attard, et al., 2009; Meng, et al., 2006; Meng, et al., 2004).

CTC are extremely rare in most patients: 1-10/7.5 ml of blood (Allard et al., 2004), among about 50 million leukocytes and 50 billion erythrocytes within that volume. For accurate characterization of the CTC it is thus of utmost importance that no cell loss is incurred and the error in the interpretation of the results is kept to a minimum. The CellSearch® system is the only clinically validated system for counting CTC (Allard, et al., 2004; Kagan et al., 2002). It is based firstly on immunomagnetic enrichment of the blood sample using antibodies directed against the epithelial cell adhesion molecule (EpCAM). A second step consists of labeling the enriched sample with fluorescent dyes for the nucleus and cytokeratins 8, 18, and 19; CD45 labeling to recognize leukocytes. In a third step, fluorescence images are recorded of the enriched and labeled sample. CTC candidates are presented to a trained reviewer who distinguishes CTC from debris and leukocytes. Limitation of the CellSearch system is that only CTC expressing both EpCAM and CK8, 18 and or 19 will be detected.

Recently, we have developed a semi-automated method for FISH analysis of CTC after they have been identified by the CellSearch™ system. Interpretation of FISH results is however encumbered by apoptosis of CTC, which is observed frequently. In addition, counting of FISH dots can be tiring and subjective, and thus likely results in differences in intra-reviewer and inter-reviewer interpretation. Automation of counting of these FISH signals -termed FISH dots hereafter- could resolve these challenges. Other work has been done in the field of automated counting of FISH dots: on cell lines (Netten et al., 1997), blood from healthy individuals (de Solorzano et al., 1998), cells from amniotic fluid (Lerner et al., 2001), and on tissue (Raimondo et al., 2005). An excellent overview of methods is available (Restif, 2006). However, to our knowledge, automated dot counting has never been applied in samples containing containing CTC. The nuclei and dots of these cells are extremely heterogeneous in shape and intensity, and therefore difficult to score, even by reviewers. Therefore, we investigated the error in counting FISH dots, and evaluated different methods to count the FISH dots by a computer algorithm.

2. Method

2.1 Patient samples

A prospective multicenter clinical trial that evaluated the utility of counting CTC for predicting response to therapy, progression-free survival, and overall survival in metastatic castration-resistant prostate cancer patients was conducted (de Bono, et al., 2008). A total of 65 clinical centers throughout the United States and Europe participated in this study after formal institutional review board approval. All patients were required to provide written informed consent. Blood was collected before starting a new treatment and at monthly intervals prior to the next cycle of therapy.

2.2 Sample preparation for CTC enumeration

Blood samples were drawn into 10 mL evacuated blood draw tubes, maintained at room temperature, and processed within 96 hours of collection. The CellSearch System (Veridex LLC, Raritan, NJ) consists of the CellTracks Autoprep®, CellTracks Magnest®, CellSearch Epithelial Cell Kit and the CellTracks Analyzer II®. The CellSearch™ Epithelial Cell Kit contains: -ferrofluids labeled with the epithelial cell adhesion molecule (EpCAM); -staining reagents 4′,2-diamidino-2-phenylindole, (DAPI), CD45-Allophycocyan (CD45-APC), cytokeratin 8, 18 Phycoerythrin, cytokeratin 19 Phycoerythrin (CK-PE); buffers to enhance cell capture (Rao et al., 2005), cell permeabilization and cell fixation. The CellTracks Autoprep immuno-magnetically enriches cells expressing EpCAM from 7.5 ml of blood, fluorescently labels the enriched cells with DAPI, CD45-APC and CK-PE, and re-suspends the cells in the cartridge placed in the CellTracks Magnest. The design of the magnets guides the magnetically labeled cells to the analysis surface (Tibbe et al., 2002).

2.3 Data acquisition for CTC enumeration

The CellTracks Magnest containing the cartridge is placed on the CellTracks Analyzer II a semi-automated fluorescence-based microscopy system that acquires images using a 10X/0.45NA objective with filters for DAPI, FITC, PE, and APC to cover the complete surface area of the cartridge. The CellSearch software identifies objects staining with DAPI and PE in the same location and generates images for the DAPI, FITC, PE, and APC filters. A reviewer selects the CTC defined as nucleated DAPI+ cells larger than 4 μm, lacking CD45-APC and expressing CK-PE from the gallery of objects, which are tabulated by the computer. Figure 1 shows an overview of the image acquisition and identification of CTC. After a scan, the cartridges were stored at room temperature until the reviewer was finished reviewing the images. Accuracy, precision, linearity, and reproducibility of the CellSearch system have been described elsewhere (Allard, et al., 2004).

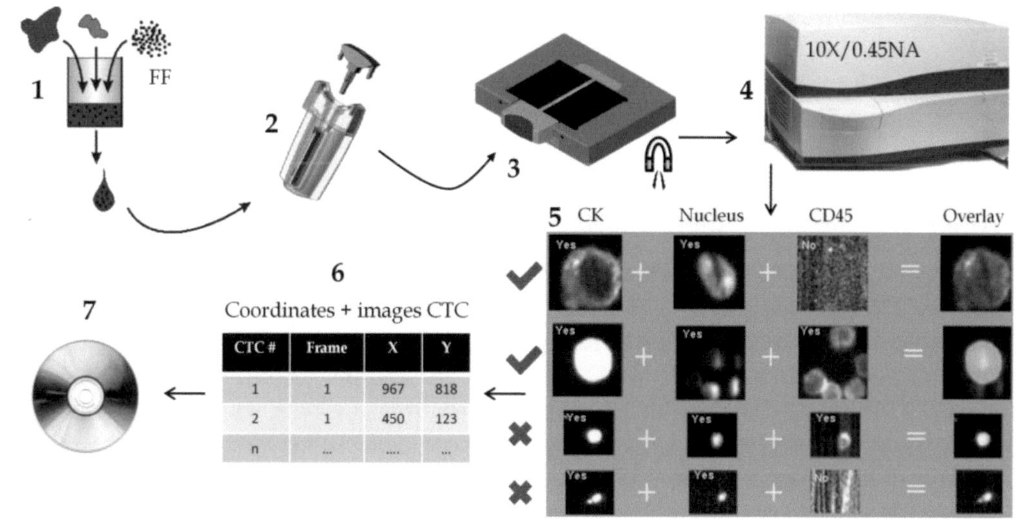

Fig. 1. Image acquisition in CellSearch. 1) Ferrofluid and staining reagents are added to the blood sample. 2) After immuno-magnetic enrichment and fluorescent labeling, the sample is inserted in a cartridge. 3) The cartridge is inserted into a Magnest to distribute the labeled cells over the analysis surface. 4) The cartridge is scanned at 10X in the CellTracks Analyzer. 5) CK+ DAPI+ objects are presented to the reviewer for CTC selection. 6) Coordinates of selected CTC are collected. 7) The coordinates and images from the scan are saved on a CD or DVD.

2.4 Samples used for FISH counting algorithm development

For algorithm development, images from cells of a patient in which no CTC were detected were used. Leukocytes which were non-specifically carried over during the CTC enrichment procedure were used as targets for this purpose, as in these cells almost no chromosomal aberrations are present and each cell should therefore contain two copies of each chromosome and gene region. The sample was labeled with a centromere specific FISH probe for chromosome 17 and a probe identifying the HER2 gene region. The centromere probe is larger than the HER2 probe, thus a difference in automated count could be expected. For the validation of the algorithm, CTC from 47 patients with hormone refractory metastatic prostate cancer labeled with probes identifying the centromeres of chromosome 1, 7, 8 and 17 were used (Swennenhuis, et al., 2009).

2.5 Sample preparation for FISH probes on CTC

Cartridges containing CTC were used for the FISH procedure. To preserve the location of the CTC for future interrogation the buffer inside the cartridge was carefully aspirated aspirated to avoid cell cell movement and replaced with methanol acetic acid. After fixation the cartridges are dried using a forced forced air flow flow and processed for FISH or stored at -20 °C for later use. FISH probes specific for the centromeric regions of chromosome 1, 7, 8, and 17 labeled with PlatinumBright-647, -550, -505, and -415, respectively, were used in this study (Kreatech, Amsterdam, The Netherlands). The probe mixture consisted of 50 μL of hybridization buffer (50% Formamide / 1 x SSC / 10% Dextran Sulfate) containing FISH probes against 1, 7, 8, and 17 at 2 ng/µL each. The cartridges were placed on a 80°C hotplate for 2 min, with the glass facing towards the hotplate, and hybridized at 42°C for 16 h. After hybridization the cartridge was washed with PBS containing DAPI (use abbreviation instead of whole word) as a nuclear counter stain.

2.6 Data acquisition for FISH probe detection in CTC

After hybridizing the FISH probes, the samples were scanned on a modified CellTracks Analyzer II. This analyzer is equipped with a 40X/0.63NA objective, to improve the resolution and light collection of the fluorescent FISH dots, and filter cubes to detect DAPI, Platinum*Bright*-647, -550, -505, and 415. The locations and images of the CTC identified in the initial 10X scan -described in 2.3- were loaded from a CD. A software program was written to move to the locations of interest and record Z-stacks to capture signals at a range of depths of the objects of interest (Swennenhuis, et al., 2009). The DAPI signals are used to correlate the 40X with the 10X scan, thereby verifying if the CTC location is correct. This was necessary, as the cells could shift up to ~200 µm due to the FISH protocol. The image acquisition procedure for the FISH probe detection is shown in figure 2.

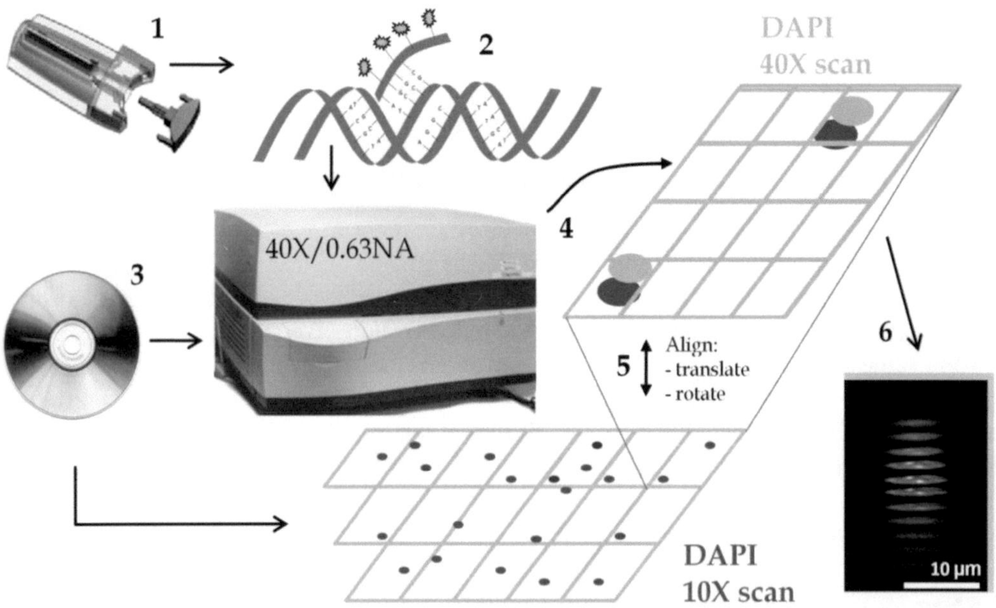

Fig. 2. Procedure for FISH probe imaging. 1) The cartridge is re-opened to carefully aspirate buffer and fixate the cells. 2) FISH reagents are added and the sample is hybridized for 16h. 3) Coordinates and images from previously assigned CTC are loaded from a CD. 4) The modified CellTracks records DAPI images at 40X at the designated coordinates and surroundings. 5) Cross correlation is performed between the DAPI images from the 40X and 10X scan to verify the correct location of the CTC. 6) After the right location is found, the FISH z-stacks are recorded.

2.7 Algorithm for counting FISH signals in leukocytes and CTC

Maximum intensity profiles were created of all the Z-stacks to speed up the counting process for human reviewing. The algorithm to identify the nucleus and count the FISH probes within this nucleus consists of five general steps:

1. enhancement and segmentation of the outline of the nucleus;
2. enhancement and segmentation of potential FISH objects;
3. exclusion of objects that are too noisy;
4. measurement of intensity and morphological features of the potential objects;
5. exclusion of objects that do not meet inclusion criteria.

Nuclei were located in the DAPI image, which was enhanced using a zero-crossing filter in combination with a gradient magnitude filter (Verbeek & Vanvliet, 1994). Edges were enhanced using a morphological gradient magnitude filter. The image of this filter was multiplied by an image filtered by a laplace-plus-dgg filter. This filter created a combination of second order derivatives in x and y, and combined it with an image of the second derivative in the direction of the maximum gradient. The combined image of the two filters is thresholded using a fixed threshold. On the outline of objects larger than 2000 pixels a distance transform was applied: every outline pixel value is replaced by its closest distance to the edge of the outline. This procedure was then followed by a watershed transform, to verify if the outline consisted of multiple maxima and were thus two or more closely spaced objects. Figure 3 shows how a distance transform improves the watershed transform in case of saturated DAPI signals. The nucleus that was at least 250 pixels in size and located closest to the middle of the image was selected as the final outline: only objects inside this outline are considered for FISH dot counting.

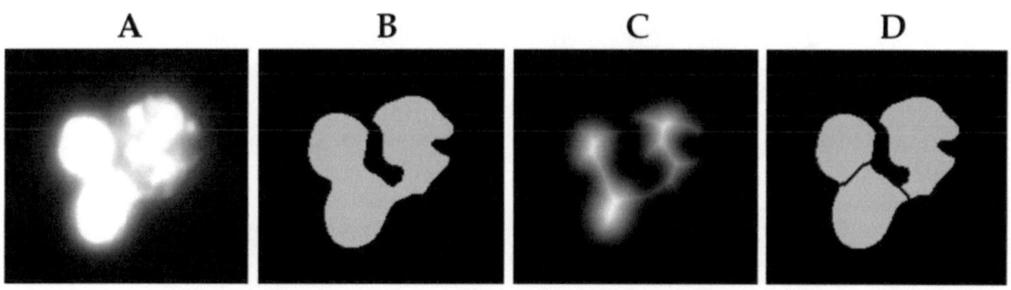

Fig. 3. Example of a distance transform aiding the watershed transform. Panel A shows the original DAPI image containing three nuclei which is thresholded to give the outline at panel B. This outline is difficult to watershed due to saturation in the original image. The distance transform shown in panel C creates a new input for the watershed transform, which successfully separates the nuclei as is shown in panel D.

In a next step, dot-like structures were enhanced. Usually this is performed by employing a tophat filter (Netten, et al., 1997). We used a method termed multiscale product (Vermolen et al., 2008) because it appeared better suited to deal with the heterogeneity of the shapes of the FISH probes. This filter increases the intensity of objects in a range of radii, using a multiplication of Gaussian kernels with different σ (ranging from 1.5 to 3.0 pixels):

$$G_{product} = (G - G_0) \cdot (G_0 - G_1) \cdot (G_1 - G_2) \tag{1}$$

with the 2D Gaussian kernel defined as

$$G(\sigma_i) = \frac{1}{2\pi\sigma_i^2} e^{-\frac{x^2+y^2}{2\sigma_i^2}} \tag{2}$$

Using a range of Gaussian kernel sizes improves robustness to variations in size of the objects of interest, compared to using a single kernel size as is done in the tophat transform method. After applying the multiscale product, objects were thresholded using the triangle threshold (Zack et al., 1977) which was multiplied by a factor of 0.1 to include all relevant dot-like structures, bright or dim. This thresholding method uses the intensity histogram of the image and is especially suited for images with few object pixels. After thresholding, a final verification was performed to exclude objects that are too noisy. The dome finding method of Restif was applied to the coordinates of the maximum of each object (Restif, 2006). This method checks nearest downhill neighbors in three level sets -up to three pixels around the maximum- and excludes objects that have more than one extra local maximum in this region. Figure 4 shows the method by which nearest downhill neighbors are checked.

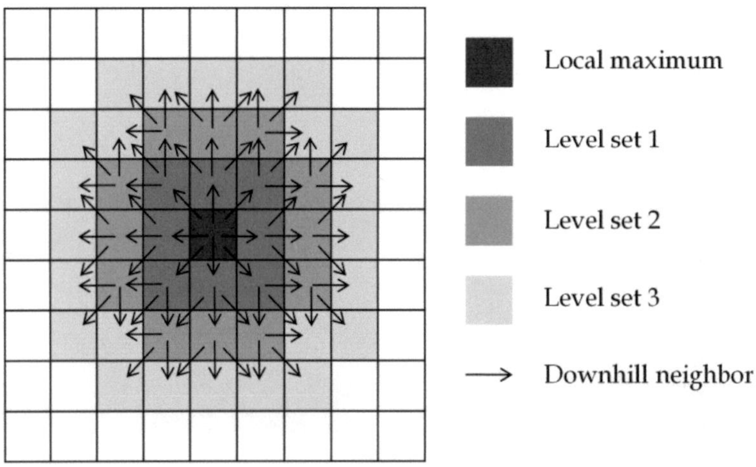

Fig. 4. Scheme for checking downhill neighbors. By checking objects in this way only dome shape objects are included. (adapted from (Restif, 2006))

Restif et al. determined that if one extra local maximum is allowed, at least 75% of the downhill neighbors should have a lower intensity. We allow one extra local maximum to include very closely spaced FISH dots. In this way, noisy objects are excluded, whether or not this noise is originating from a high or low intensity background. Finally, measurements were performed on these objects: size, maximum intensity, mean intensity, total intensity, relative intensity, roundness, and perimeter were saved for every object. Relative intensity was defined as the total intensity of the object related to the total intensity of the brightest object within the same nucleus. Using these measurements, different exclusion criteria were tested. Combinations of measurements were tested on the leukocyte training set to exclude debris and keep the true FISH dots. Figure 5 gives a schematic overview of the procedure.

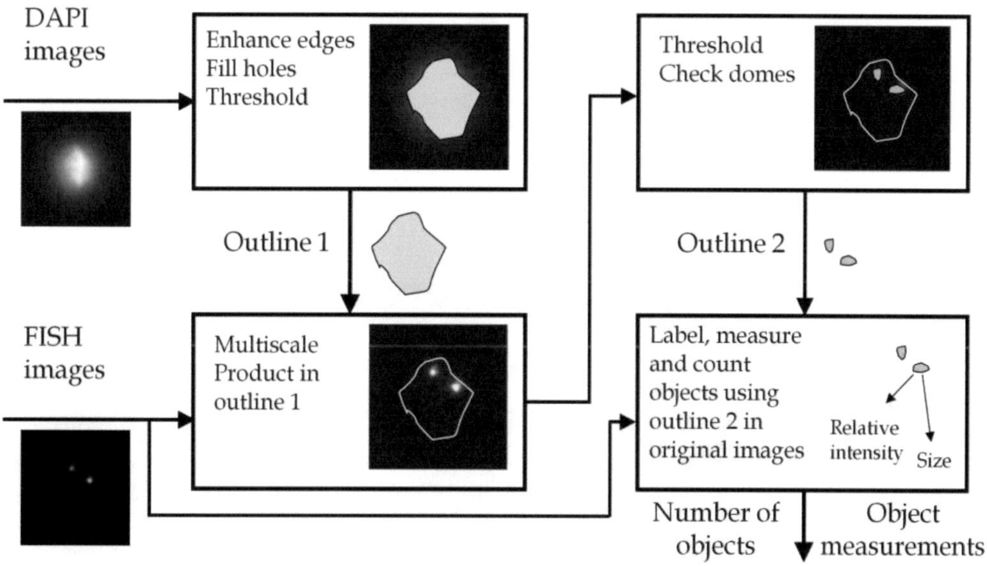

Fig. 5. Schematic representation of the counting process. DAPI images are loaded and their outline is determined. Within this outline, a multiscale product is applied. Objects within outline 1 are thresholded and checked for dome-like structures. Finally, the objects are counted and measured.

2.8 Expert reviewing of samples

Next to the algorithm, five expert reviewers counted FISH probe signals in the leukocytes, using a macro written in the program ImageJ (Collins, 2007). They reviewed the set two times: the first time they were asked to review all images, the second time they could skip images that were unclear in their view. In this way it could be measured how sure reviewers were. All CTC samples were also reviewed by the five expert reviewers.

3. Results

492 leukocytes and 500 CTC were imaged by the modified CellTracks Analyzer II. Figure 6 shows an example of a FISH Z-stack from a leukocyte in top and slice view, from which a maximum profile was created. The profiles were processed by the algorithm, requiring ~2 minutes for each sample and counted by human reviewers, requiring ~2 hours for each sample. Figure 7 shows the different steps of the algorithm: segmentation of the nucleus, enhancement of dot-like structures and the final outline of nucleus and the dots.

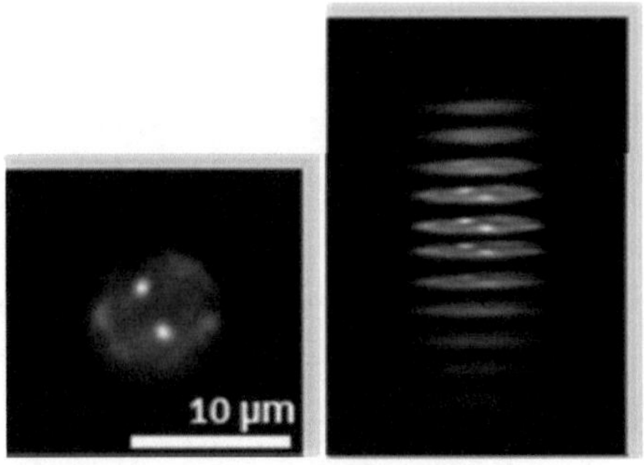

Fig. 6. Example of a recorded Z-stack of FISH probes in a leukocyte in top-view, panel A, and in slice-view, panel B. Distance between the slices is 1 μm

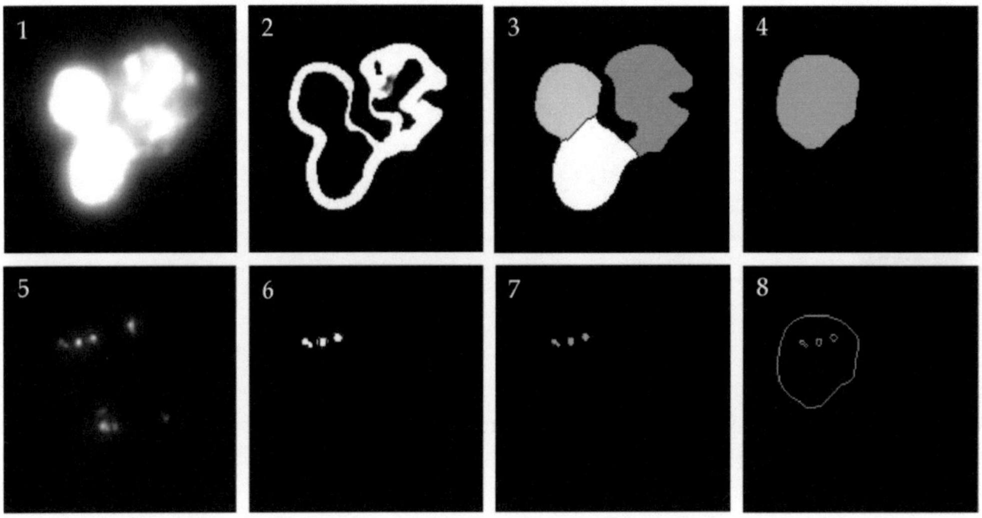

Fig. 7. Example of the image processing steps on a recorded DAPI and FISH image. 1) original DAPI image; 2) edge enhanced DAPI image; 3) outline after thresholding and watershed; 4) final DAPI outline; 5) original FISH image; 6) FISH image after multiscale product; 7) outline FISH image; 8) final outlines of DAPI and FISH.

3.1 Counting of the leukocyte training sample

After comparison of the manual and automated counts in the training sample, it became apparent that only the measurements "size" and "relative intensity" had a positive impact on the counting efficiency of the algorithm. After objects were measured and counted in the HER2 channel the objects, with a relative intensity lower than 30% of the brightest dot, within that nucleus were excluded. For the centromere 17 channel this threshold was optimal at 25%. Objects smaller than 5 pixels were also excluded. Automatic counting of chromosomes in leukocytes resulted in an accuracy of 97.8% of the HER2 dots and 97.5% of the centromere 17 dots. Accurate here means "equal to the manual count of the subset of images were all reviewers agreed upon" (n=409 for HER2 and n=347 for centromere 17). The mean inter-reviewer agreement was 92.6%±2.3% and 91.7%±1.7% and the mean intra-reviewer agreement was 96.5%±2.7% and 97.0%±1.8% for the HER2 and centromere 17 probes, respectively. Table 1 gives an overview of the counting efficiencies after review of HER2 and centromere 17 of the whole data set and the data set containing only the images with objects that could be easily identified by the reviewer, compared with the count generated by the algorithm. In figure 8 the distribution of the count of the PC and five reviewers are shown. The count of the reviewers is represented by the mean and the standard deviation for each chromosome count.

HER2	Rev 1	Rev 2	Rev 3	Rev 4	Rev 5	PC
Rev 1	96.2%±1.7%	91.3%±2.5%	93.9%±2.1%	93.5%±2.2%	95.5%±1.9%	90.3%±2.6%
Rev 2	91.3%±2.5%	92.5%±2.3%	89.9%±2.7%	89.3%±2.7%	90.9%±2.6%	85.0%±3.2%
Rev 3	93.9%±2.2%	91.0%±2.6%	95.7%±1.8%	92.7%±2.3%	96.0%±1.8%	90.5%±2.6%
Rev 4	98.7%±1.2%	97.7%±1.6%	97.9%±1.5%	99.2%±1.0%	92.9%±2.3%	87.6%±2.9%
Rev 5	97.3%±1.5%	93.0%±2.3%	96.2%±1.8%	99.2%±1.0%	98.9%±1.0%	92.1%±2.4%
PC	90.5%±2.6%	87.4%±2.9%	89.8%±2.7%	96.9%±1.8%	92.6%±2.4%	100.0%-0.4%
Cent17						
Rev 1	96.4%±1.7%	92.9%±2.3%	92.7%±2.3%	93.7%±2.2%	90.5%±2.6%	87.6%±2.9%
Rev 2	92.3%±2.4%	94.9%±2.0%	93.9%±2.1%	90.7%±2.6%	92.3%±2.4%	88.1%±2.9%
Rev 3	95.0%±2.0%	94.5%±2.1%	96.0%±1.8%	90.3%±2.6%	91.7%±2.5%	85.4%±3.1%
Rev 4	96.1%±1.9%	98.3%±1.3%	97.0%±1.7%	99.0%±1.0%	88.5%±2.8%	89.1%±2.8%
Rev 5	96.0%±1.9%	96.0%±1.9%	98.1%±1.4%	96.4%±1.9%	98.6%±1.2%	88.5%±2.8%
PC	87.4%±2.9%	91.5%±2.5%	88.4%±2.9%	95.4%±2.1%	91.7%±2.7%	100.0%-0.4%

Table 1. Agreement between expert reviewers and the PC algorithm when reviewing leukocytes. In the upper right part of the table (white), the agreement of the first review is shown in which the reviewer had to review the full dataset (n=492). Second, in the lower left part of the table (dark grey) the agreement of the second review is shown, in which the reviewers only reviewed the cells they were certain of (the "obvious" dataset). Last, the intra-reviewer variation is given on the diagonal of the table (light grey).

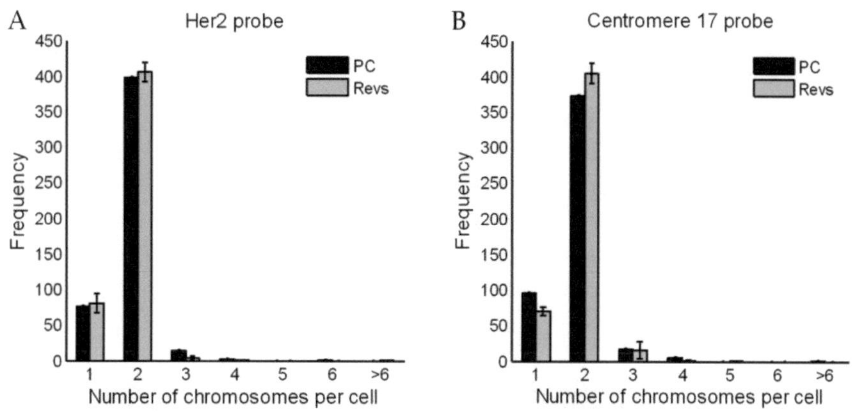

Fig. 8. Number of leukocytes for the HER2 gene probe (panel A) and the centromere of chromosome 17 probe (panel B) as counted by the PC and the five reviewers (n=492).

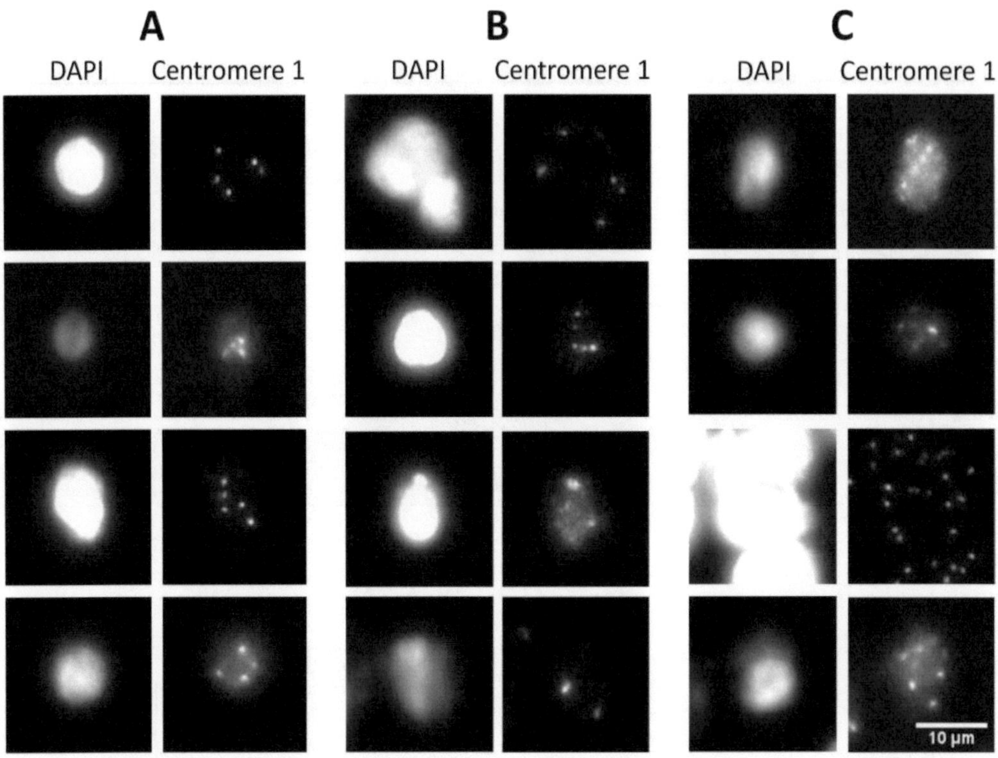

Fig. 9. Example of FISH images. Panel A shows cases were all reviewers and the PC agreed. Panel B shows examples were all the human reviewers agreed, but the PC disagreed on the number of FISH dots. Panel C shows examples with the largest discrepancy among reviewers.

3.2 Counting of a sample containing CTC

After processing a sample containing CTC it became clear that the threshold for relative intensity was strongly related to the quality of the FISH probe used, and thus probe dependent. Slight adjustment of the relative intensity criteria to a range from 14%-20% was necessary to ensure reasonable counting by the algorithm. This value was correlated with the average of the maximum intensity of all the objects in a channel: if this average was high, then the relative intensity should be set lower. Figure 9 shows three categories of examples from the data set: panel A shows examples were all the reviewers and the PC agreed; panel B shows examples were all reviewers agreed, *but the PC did not;* finally, panel C shows examples where there was a large discrepancy between all reviewers and the PC.

Agreement of the PC with the subset of cells on which all reviewers agreed was 76.1% (n=238), 83.9% (n=280), 86.6% (n=209), and 85.3% (n=251) for probes from centromere 1, 7, 8, and 17 respectively. Mean inter-reviewer agreement was 70.9%, 75.3%, 66.8%, and 72.3% for these four channels. Figure 10 show the agreement between all reviewers in detail and the histogram of the count.

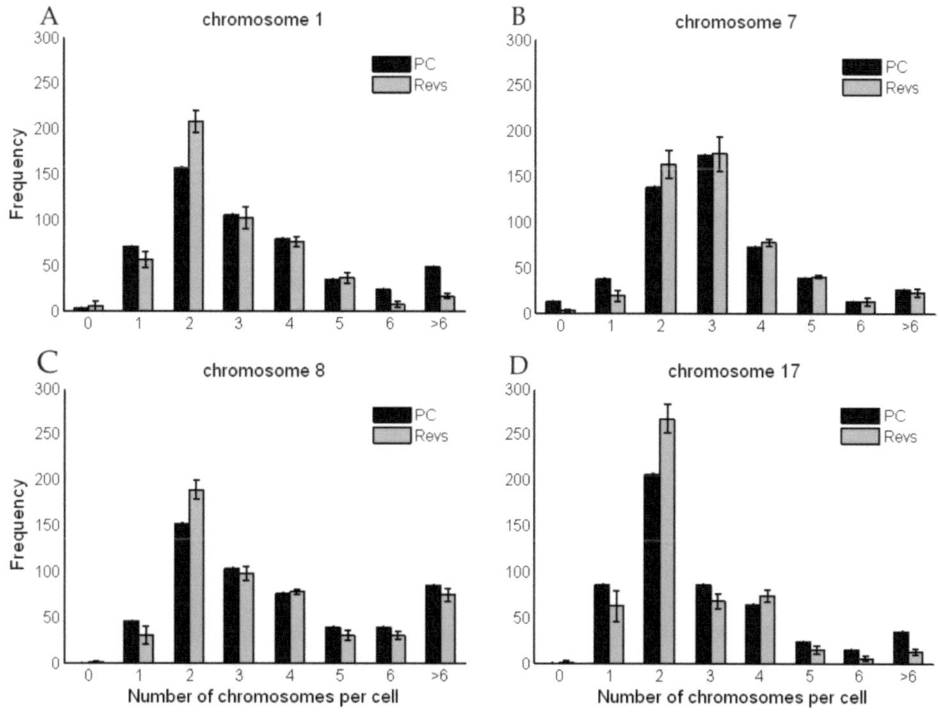

Fig. 10. Number of CTC containing 0-6 or >6 dots for the centromere of chromosomes 1,7,8, and 17 probe (panel A-D) as counted by the PC and the five reviewers (n=500). The reviewer count is given as the mean of the frequency of each number and its standard deviation.

4. Conclusion

4.1 Automated counting is necessary and feasible

We have shown that reliable automated counting of FISH probes on EpCAM+DAPI+CK+CD45- cells is both necessary and feasible. Comparing expert reviews revealed that intra-reviewer variation -the same expert reviewing a data set twice- could be as high as 3.5% of the cells. Inter-reviewer variation was higher: 7.5%; these numbers were both acquired for the "easy" leukocyte samples with low copy numbers. Variation between reviewers while reviewing CTC samples could be as high as 33.2% (centromere chromosome 8), showing that the number of signals in a nucleus is of great influence on counting accuracy, as is the knowledge of the reviewer that he or she is dealing with CTC or leukocytes. Furthermore, reviewing 500 FISH nuclei in four channels takes several hours, while the computer only needs a few minutes.

From the results it becomes clear that review of chromosome 1 and 8 was the most difficult, for both PC and reviewer. These probes had on average a factor two lower intensities than the probes from chromosomes 7 and 17. Thus, the inter-reviewer agreement was lower as well as the agreement with the PC. The dome finding part of the algorithm revealed the same: it removed objects that were too noisy in 17% and 13% of the nuclei in the channel from chromosome 1 and 8 respectively, and only in 8% of the nuclei from channels of chromosome 7 and 17. Signal to noise ratios were clearly lower in channels were the agreement was lower.

4.2 Sources of error for human and PC

Agreement between PC and reviewer was good when control samples were reviewed, and reasonable when CTC were reviewed. The difference between the two data sets could be attributed to a few main sources of error:

1. Nuclei were well separated in the leukocyte sample, the CTC samples contained more clusters. While these clusters are usually easily resolved by eye, the algorithm had more difficulty in this task. Figure 9, panel B shows an example in row 1: two closely spaced nuclei with almost saturated intensity. In this case the signals of the nuclei are close to saturation and although a distance transform and watershed transform was applied, they were still segmented as one. The PC thus over-counted in this example.
2. Because the DAPI signal from the nuclei can vary greatly between samples, some signals fall just outside the segmented outline of the nucleus as determined by the algorithm. This is the case when the signal from the nucleus is relatively dim, as is shown in figure 9, panel B, row 4, where the reviewers counted two probes and the PC counted only one. This challenge could be resolved by dilating the outline nuclei more than is done now. However, closely spaced nuclei will be resolved worse in this case. The heterogeneity of the shape and size of the nucleus is largely due to presence of ferrofluid in combination with the fixation step in the FISH procedure. The ferrofluid particles were added to keep the cells tightly located to the imaging surface. However, due to the influence of these magnetic particles and the tendency of some cells to adhere to surfaces, the DNA spreads over the surface. Ferrofluid particles that line up under influence of the magnetic field force these cells to spread even further. Thus in the DAPI images even small islands of DNA were visible, that clearly were part of a bigger nucleus, making it more difficult for the algorithm to measure a perfect outline of the nucleus and include all the DNA in the dot counting. Figure 11 shows an example of this effect.

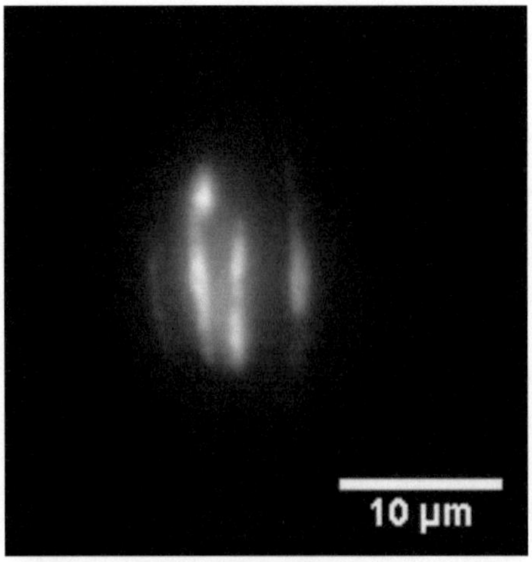

Fig. 11. Example of a nucleus spread due to fixation of the cell. Note the vertical lines that were created by ferrofluid aggregates that follow the local magnetic field. This type of nucleus is especially difficult to segment correctly.

3. The CTC sample had a larger variety in signal quality. Although the segmentation algorithm is dynamic on the histogram, it is still difficult for the PC to distinguish between what a reviewer calls a "true signal" and debris. For example, when a reviewer sees two signals -a bright and a relatively dim one-, he or she will usually count two. However, when five bright signals and one dim signal are seen, the dim object is more often neglected. Figure 9 panel B rows 2 and 3 show examples of difference in counting because of relative intensity. In row 2, the reviewers counted five and the pc four, while in row three, the reviewers counted two and the PC three probes. The PC counts 100% reproducible, but does not take into account these human considerations. For this analysis, it is thus very difficult to get an absolute "golden truth".
4. It still is hard for the PC to distinguish between a split probe (one chromosome that had two signals) and two closely spaced chromosomes. It is however not known how often a reviewer misclassifies such an object. A reviewer can structurally ignore or assign the split spots. The PC cannot and counts these items according to the algorithm. The number of cells that have these split spots may vary between samples and also within samples (e.g. between lymphocyte and CTC). The PC might not be able to distinguish between these, but if this factor appears to be of influence to the result, the PC could use the measurements of the probes -i.e. relative intensity coupled to size of closely spaced probes- to estimate the probability of these splits in the cells. Leukocytes could be used as an internal control for measuring the frequency of these splits and for estimating a relevant "size/relative intensity" threshold.

The above error sources may seem a big challenge, but are not of importance for the clinical relevant observations, which is the presence or absence of aneuploidy to ascertain the cancerous origin of the cells and the presence of amplification or deletions of specific genes that may be used to guide certain therapies. CTC are very heterogeneous: within one patient a wide variety of chromosomal aberrations could be spotted. So whether or not a certain cell has five or six copies is of lesser importance than the fact that this number is greater than two. When comparing counts that are greater than two or not, the reviewer and PC concur in 87%, 93%, 94%, and 94% of the cells for centromere 1, 7, 8, and 17 respectively for the data set in which all reviewers agree. This demonstrates that in about 90% of the cases, the PC and reviewer will draw the same conclusion about the ploidy status of the cells identified as tumor cells.

Figure 9 panel C shows examples in which the reviewers greatly disagreed. Two examples of varying signal intensities (rows 1 and 2) and two examples of difficulty of locating the true outline of the nucleus (row 3 en 4) are given. It could be argued that the example of row 1 isn't suitable for reviewing at all because the background staining is too high. For reviewers, there is no real quantitative criterion whether or not to reject a certain object based on its intensity distribution. However, the PC has such a criterion: it can easily check if a maximum of an object is surrounded by more than two other local maxima. If this is the case, then an object should be excluded. We perform this verification by means of the dome finding function. In this way, the PC performs more reliable than the human reviewers.

4.3 Future research

In the future, the algorithm may be optimized further by using clinical data. When coupling for instance response to a therapy of a patient to the aberration of the genes in the CTC the treatment is targeting, a better golden truth may be found. Furthermore, quality of FISH could still be improved. Split probes are still a big challenge for the PC, but also for establishing a good count by reviewers. Consequently a quality score could be set by the algorithm by measuring intensity variations, for instance in carried-over leukocytes. This score could be used as an internal control in each patient sample to adjust exclusion criteria and to reject cells that are not suitable for interpretation. Finally, removal of ferrofluid could greatly improve the segmentation of the nucleus. Aggregation of ferrofluid particles disturbs the natural shape of the nucleus and blocks a fraction of the fluorescence light. Implementation of physical filters to enrich CTC by size would not require any ferrofluid and could be an improvement in the next generation tumor cell capturing devices.

5. Acknowledgments

We would like to acknowledge Ronald Sipkema for his contribution to the software for the improved CellTracks Analyzer.

6. References

Allard, W. J.; Matera, J.; Miller, M. C.; Repollet, M.; Connelly, M. C.; Rao, C.; Tibbe, A. G. J.; Uhr, J. W. & Terstappen, L. (2004). Tumor cells circulate in the peripheral blood of all major carcinomas but not in healthy subjects or patients with nonmalignant diseases, *Clinical Cancer Research,* Vol.10, No.20, (Oct 2004), pp. 6897-6904, ISSN 1078-0432

Attard, G.; Swermenhuis, J. F.; Olmos, D.; Reid, A. H. M.; Vickers, E.; A'Hern, R.; Levink, R.; Coumans, F.; Moreira, J.; Riisnaes, R.; Oommen, N. B.; Hawche, G.; Jameson, C.; Thompson, E.; Sipkema, R.; Carden, C. P.; Parker, C.; Dearnaley, D.; Kaye, S. B.; Cooper, C. S.; Molina, A.; Cox, M. E.; Terstappen, L. & de Bono, J. S. (2009). Characterization of ERG, AR and PTEN Gene Status in Circulating Tumor Cells from Patients with Castration-Resistant Prostate Cancer, *Cancer Research,* Vol.69, No.7, (Apr 2009), pp. 2912-2918, ISSN 0008-5472

Cohen, S. J.; Punt, C. J. A.; Iannotti, N.; Saidman, B. H.; Sabbath, K. D.; Gabrail, N. Y.; Picus, J.; Morse, M.; Mitchell, E.; Miller, M. C.; Doyle, G. V.; Tissing, H.; Terstappen, L. & Meropol, N. J. (2008). Relationship of circulating tumor cells to tumor response, progression-free survival, and overall survival in patients with metastatic colorectal cancer, *Journal of Clinical Oncology,* Vol.26, No.19, 2008), pp. 3213-3221, ISSN 0732-183X

Collins, T. J. (2007). ImageJ for microscopy, *Biotechniques,* Vol.43, No.1, (Jul 2007), pp. 25-+, ISSN 0736-6205

Cristofanilli, M.; Budd, G. T.; Ellis, M. J.; Stopeck, A.; Matera, J.; Miller, M. C.; Reuben, J. M.; Doyle, G. V.; Allard, W. J.; Terstappen, L. & Hayes, D. F. (2004). Circulating tumor cells, disease progression, and survival in metastatic breast cancer, *New England Journal of Medicine,* Vol.351, No.8, (Aug 2004), pp. 781-791, ISSN 0028-4793

de Bono, J. S.; Attard, G.; Adjei, A.; Pollak, M. N.; Fong, P. C.; Haluska, P.; Roberts, L.; Melvin, C.; Repollet, M.; Chianese, D.; Connely, M.; Terstappen, L. & Gualberto, A. (2007). Potential applications for circulating tumor cells expressing the insulin-like growth factor-I receptor, *Clinical Cancer Research,* Vol.13, No.12, (Jun 2007), pp. 3611-3616, ISSN 1078-0432 de Bono, J. S.; Scher, H. I.; Montgomery, R. B.; Parker, C.; Miller, M. C.; Tissing, H.; Doyle, G. V.; Terstappen, L.; Pienta, K. J. & Raghavan, D. (2008). Circulating Tumor Cells Predict Survival Benefit from Treatment in Metastatic Castration-Resistant Prostate Cancer, *Clinical Cancer Research,* Vol.14, No.19, (Oct 2008), pp. 6302-6309, ISSN 1078-0432

de Solorzano, C. O.; Santos, A.; Vallcorba, I.; Garcia-Sagredo, J. M. & del Pozo, F. (1998). Automated FISH spot counting in interphase nuclei: Statistical validation and data correction, *Cytometry,* Vol.31, No.2, (Feb 1 1998), pp. 93-99, ISSN

Fehm, T.; Sagalowsky, A.; Clifford, E.; Beitsch, P.; Saboorian, H.; Euhus, D.; Meng, S. D.; Morrison, L.; Tucker, T.; Lane, N.; Ghadimi, B. M.; Heselmeyer-Haddad, K.; Ried, T.; Rao, C. & Uhr, J. (2002). Cytogenetic evidence that circulating epithelial cells in patients with carcinoma are malignant, *Clinical Cancer Research,* Vol.8, No.7, (Jul 2002), pp. 2073-2084, ISSN 1078-0432

Hayes, D. F.; Walker, T. M.; Singh, B.; Vitetta, E. S.; Uhr, J. W.; Gross, S.; Rao, C.; Doyle, G. V. & Terstappen, L. (2002). Monitoring expression of HER-2 on circulating epithelial cells in patients with advanced breast cancer, *International Journal of Oncology,* Vol.21, No.5, (Nov 2002), pp. 1111-1117, ISSN 1019-6439

Kagan, M.; Howard, D.; Bendele, T.; Mayes, J.; Silvia, J.; Repollet, M.; Doyle, J.; Allard, J.; Tu, N.; Bui, T.; Russell, T.; Rao, C.; Hermann, M.; Rutner, H. & Terstappen, L. (2002). A sample preparation and analysis system for identification of circulating tumor cells, *Journal of Clinical Ligand Assay,* Vol.25, No.1, (Spr 2002), pp. 104-110, ISSN 1081-1672

Lerner, B.; Clocksin, W. F.; Dhanjal, S.; Hulten, M. A. & Bishop, C. M. (2001). Automatic signal classification in fluorescence in situ hybridization images, *Cytometry,* Vol.43, No.2, (Feb 1 2001), pp. 87-93, ISSN 0196-4763

Meng, S.; Tripathy, D.; Shete, S.; Ashfaq, R.; Saboorian, H.; Haley, B.; Frenkel, E.; Euhus, D.; Leitch, M.; Osborne, C.; Clifford, E.; Perkins, S.; Beitsch, P.; Khan, A.; Morrison, L.; Herlyn, D.; Terstappen, L.; Lane, N.; Wang, J. & Uhr, J. (2006). uPAR and HER-2 gene status in individual breast cancer cells from blood and tissues, *Proceedings Of The National Academy Of Sciences Of The United States Of America,* Vol.103, No.46, (Nov 2006), pp. 17361-17365, ISSN 0027-8424

Meng, S. D.; Tripathy, D.; Shete, S.; Ashfaq, R.; Haley, B.; Perkins, S.; Beitsch, P.; Khan, A.; Euhus, D.; Osborne, C.; Frenkel, E.; Hoover, S.; Leitch, M.; Clifford, E.; Vitetta, E.; Morrison, L.; Herlyn, D.; Terstappen, L.; Fleming, T.; Fehm, T.; Tucker, T.; Lane, N.; Wang, J. Q. & Uhr, J. (2004). HER-2 gene amplification can be acquired as breast cancer progresses, *Proceedings Of The National Academy Of Sciences Of The United States Of America,* Vol.101, No.25, (Jun 2004), pp. 9393-9398, ISSN 0027-8424

Netten, H.; Young, I. T.; vanVliet, L. J.; Tanke, H. J.; Vroljik, H. & Sloos, W. C. R. (1997). FISH and chips: Automation of fluorescent dot counting in interphase cell nuclei, *Cytometry,* Vol.28, No.1, (May 1 1997), pp. 1-10, ISSN 0196-4763

Raimondo, F.; Gavrielides, M. A.; Karayannopoulou, G.; Lyroudia, K.; Pitas, I. & Kostopoulos, I. (2005). Automated evaluation of Her-2/neu status in breast tissue from fluorescent in situ hybridization images, *Ieee Transactions On Image Processing,* Vol.14, No.9, (Sep 2005), pp. 1288-1299, ISSN 1057-7149

Rao, C. G.; Chianese, D.; Doyle, G. V.; Miller, M. C.; Russell, T.; Sanders, R. A. & Terstappen, L. (2005). Expression of epithelial cell adhesion molecule in carcinoma cells present in blood and primary and metastatic tumors, *International Journal of Oncology,* Vol.27, No.1, (Jul 2005), pp. 49-57, ISSN 1019-6439

Smirnov, D. A.; Zweitzig, D. R.; Foulk, B. W.; Miller, M. C.; Doyle, G. V.; Pienta, K. J.; Meropol, N. J.; Weiner, L. M.; Cohen, S. J.; Moreno, J. G.; Connelly, M. C.; Terstappen, L. & O'Hara, S. M. (2005). Global gene expression profiling of circulating tumor cells, *Cancer Research,* Vol.65, No.12, (Jun 2005), pp. 4993-4997, ISSN 0008-5472

Swennenhuis, J. F.; Tibbe, A. G.; Levink, R.; Sipkema, R. C. & Terstappen, L. W. (2009). Characterization of circulating tumor cells by fluorescence in situ hybridization, *Cytometry Part A,* Vol.75, No.6, (Jun 2009), pp. 520-7, ISSN 1552-4930 (Electronic)

Tibbe, A. G. J.; de Grooth, B. G.; Greve, J.; Dolan, G. J.; Rao, C. & Terstappen, L. (2002). Magnetic field design for selecting and aligning immunomagnetic labeled cells, *Cytometry,* Vol.47, No.3, (Mar 2002), pp. 163-172, ISSN 0196-4763

Verbeek, P. W. & Vanvliet, L. J. (1994). On the location error of curved edges in low-pass filtered 2-D and 3-D images, *Ieee Transactions on Pattern Analysis and Machine Intelligence,* Vol.16, No.7, (Jul 1994), pp. 726-733, ISSN 0162-8828

Vermolen, B. J.; Garini, Y.; Young, I. T.; Dirks, R. W. & Raz, V. (2008). Segmentation and analysis of the three-dimensional redistribution of nuclear components in human mesenchymal stem cells, *Cytometry Part A,* Vol.73A, No.9, (Sep 2008), pp. 816-824, ISSN 1552-4922

Zack, G. W.; Rogers, W. E. & Latt, S. A. (1977). Automatic-Measurement Of Sister Chromatid Exchange Frequency, *Journal of Histochemistry & Cytochemistry,* Vol.25, No.7, 1977), pp. 741-753, ISSN 0022-1554

8

Cytokeratin 18 (CK18) and Caspase-Cleaved CK18 (ccCK18) as Response Markers in Anticancer Therapy

Hamilton Gerhard
Ludwig Boltzmann Cluster of Translational Oncology, Vienna, Austria

1. Introduction

Novel anticancer drugs are urgently needed for treatment of many types of tumors and, therefore, appropriate response markers are required that in preclinical studies and in human phase I and phase II clinical trials allow for a rapid evaluation of their efficacy and toxicity. The current drug development in oncology is hampered by a high discontinuation rate for new agents, partly due to a lack of appropriate preclinical studies that are capable of accurately predicting clinical suitability. Since newer targeted molecular therapeutics are often cytostatic, rather than cytotoxic, assessment of tumor shrinkage as an endpoint may not be suitable to estimate efficacy (Wittenburg & Gustafson, 2011). Better tumor response markers are expected to improve the drug development process in oncology by leading to a increased comprehension of the factors determining efficacy and toxicity, and, ultimately, to fewer failures. The present work reviews the conventional methods of the assessment of the activity of chemotherapeutics and discusses the newer response markers, particularly the use of CK18 and CK18 fragments for this purpose.

2. Assessment of tumor response to anticancer agents

2.1 Clinical parameters of tumor response

In oncology, a "clinical endpoint" is defined as a characteristic or variable that reflects how a patient feels, functions, or survives, while a "surrogate end point" is defined as a biomarker that is intended to substitute for a clinical end point. The process of proving a linkage between the biomarker and a clinical end point is termed "evaluation" in preference to validation. Assessment of tumor response to therapy is necessary for evaluation of the efficacy of novel anticancer drugs in clinical trials and, furthermore, response evaluation with high individual precision may allow for individualized therapy rather than standardized treatment. The definitive proof of the effectiveness of a therapy is improvement in clinical symptoms and survival (Table 1). However, overall survival (OS) as the ultimate end point of tumor therapies has the disadvantage of the requirement of a prolonged observation period depending on the respective tumor entity. The choice of surrogate and true end points has become a much debated and critical issue in oncology. Many recent randomized trials in solid tumor oncology have used progression-free survival

(PFS) as the primary end point because it is available earlier than OS and not influenced by second-line treatments (Saad et al., 2010). PFS is now undergoing validation as a surrogate end point in various malignancies; however, in advanced breast cancer validation of PFS as a surrogate for OS has so far been unsuccessful. In advanced colorectal cancer, in contrast, current evidence indicates that PFS is a valid surrogate for OS after first-line treatment with chemotherapy.

The activity of anticancer drugs is evaluated by measuring changes in tumor size in response to treatment (Therasse et al., 2000). In the early 1980s, the World Health Organization (WHO) developed recommendations in an attempt to standardize criteria for response assessment, and these were adopted as the standard method for evaluating tumor response. Tumor size has traditionally been estimated from bidimensional measurements (the product of the longest diameter and its longest perpendicular diameter for each tumor). However, measuring in two dimensions and then calculating their products and their sums is laborious and error-prone. The changes in one diameter only are now used since this parameter relates more closely to the fixed proportion of cells killed by a standard dose of chemotherapy than do changes in the bidimensional product. The response evaluation criteria in solid tumors (RECIST) categorises response to therapy as follows: complete response (CR), the disappearance of all target lesions; partial response (PR), at least a 30% decrease in the sum of the longest diameter of all target lesions; progressive disease (PD), at least a 20% increase in the sum of the longest diameter of all target lesions or the appearance of one or more new lesions; and stable disease (SD), neither sufficient shrinkage to qualify for PR nor sufficient increase to qualify for PD (Therasse et al., 2000). Appropriateness of RECIST criteria, for example, whether the change in tumor size is a proper end point for response assessment, has been widely discussed (Paules et al., 2011).

Traditional standards may not be appropriate to assess the efficacy of emerging numbers of cytostatic agents, which do not result in tumor regression to a point of PR or CR. Proposals of a general means of assessment of both cytotoxic and cystostatic effects must be developed (Gwyther & Schwartz, 2008). Since the natural growth rates of the tumors are not considered, a specific treatment that kills the same fraction of tumor cells in two different tumor types will give different results if the proliferation rates are different (Mehrara et al., 2011). A reduction of tumor size after therapy seems to indicate a better prognosis; however, this assumption is not necessarily correct when other tumor characteristics are unfavorable. Finally, drugs that result in stable disease without an objective response may retard tumor growth sufficiently to improve patient survival. Numerous studies have shown that the effect of treatment on tumors can be assessed by means of changes in tumor characteristics other than size, for example, estimated by positron emission tomography (PET) or magnetic resonance imaging or spectroscopy (Padhani & Miles, 2010). Moreover, tumor growth rate was demonstrated to constitute a valuable parameter for survival of patients and the change in tumor growth rate can serve as a surrogate end point for determination of therapy response (Mehrara et al., 2011).

2.2 Biomarkers for assessment of tumor response

Anticancer drug development remains slow, costly and unsuccessful in many cases. Suitable biomarkers are also seen as facilitating decision making during early discovery up to the point of preclinical evaluation (Carden et al., 2010). With the growing knowledge of the human genome and genetic alterations in cancers, the development of new anticancer therapies has shifted from cytotoxic agents to mechanism-driven drugs (Zhao et al., 2009). As a result, tumor response to therapy may not be observed at the same magnitude or speed by conventional tumor imaging. Tumor-specific tracers and imaging techniques to visualize and quantify tumor changes at histologic and molecular levels aims for measuring tumor response more objectively.

Most anticancer drugs are effective only in subgroup of patients and currently accurate and reliable prediction which patient will benefit from a specific therapeutic regimen is restricted to special cases. Various techniques have, therefore, been developed for monitoring tumor response to therapy but so far measuring tumor shrinkage on computerized tomography (CT) represents the current standard (Weber, 2009). However, CT is inaccurate in differentiating viable tumor from necrotic or fibrotic tissue and limited in detecting responses in tumors that do not change in size during therapy. One way of addressing this might be the use of predictive biomarkers to select patients for Phase I/II trials. Such biomarkers, which predict response to molecular-targeted agents, have the potential to enrich the fraction of patients more likely to benefit. Forecasting of tumor response based on gene expression data is feasible in certain cases, for transcripts like HER2, KRAS, mutated EGFR and others, but gene signatures are only appropriate to give a probability of increased success or failure of specific treatment modalities (Mandrekar & Sargent, 2010; Goodison et al., 2010). A fundamental problem of using gene expression profiles or other molecular characteristics of tumor tissue to predict tumor response is the fact that malignant tumors are constantly changing and adapting to their environment. As a consequence, most responses to chemotherapy or targeted drugs are relatively short-lived and resistant cancer cells evolve quickly. Because of these inherent limitations in the current approaches for response prediction, the need for techniques to monitor tumor response to therapy well in advance of clinical parameters is obvious. Furthermore, the tests aim to identify nonresponding patients early, in order to stop ineffective therapies and avoid unnecessary exposure to side effects.

2.2.1 Serum tumor markers

The ultimate goal in drug development is to use tumor response as a surrogate for clinical benefit, because response is generally faster to assess and also less influenced by factors such as patient performance status or second-line therapy. The approach comprising serum tumor markers tries to measure specimens specifically secreted by cancer cells into the blood and their modulation by therapeutic interventions. The use of changes in serum markers as a measure of tumor response is appealing because it is noninvasive, can be repeated frequently and has a relatively low cost. Furthermore, it offers the opportunity to measure tumor response independently of the affected sites with a single parameter. To be useful the biomarker response evaluation must be in good agreement with data recorded by traditional anatomical methods. However, biomarkers that provide information about induction of tumor cell death will not necessarily correlate with clinical outcome (Linder & Alaiya, 2009).

Since the original description of carcinoembryonic antigen (CEA), a large number of tumor-associated proteins have been detected in sera from cancer patients. Clinically suitable markers to monitor disease progression include CEA, prostate-specific antigen (PSA), tissue polypeptide antigen (TPA), tissue polypeptide-specific antigen (TPS), CA19-9 and CA15-3, among others (Mishra & Verma, 2010). However, results have to be checked carefully since, for example, a decline in PSA levels may be the result of dedifferentiation of the tumor and not of a successful therapeutic modality.

In addition, proteins that are not usually secreted by tumor cells may be detected in the circulation of cancer patients. Examples of such proteins are S100B (Ghanem et al., 2001), CA125 (Beck et al., 1998), high-mobility group box protein 1 (HMGB1, Candolfi et al., 2009; Gauley & Pisetsky, 2009), CKs (Stigbrand, 2001; Linder et al., 2004) and others. Nonsecreted intracellular proteins seem to reach the circulation upon cell death. In cases of enhanced cellular turnover and cell death, such as in cancer, the local clearance mechanisms through macrophages will be overcharged and apoptotic bodies will disintegrate in a process termed secondary necrosis (Kroemer et al., 1998).

Clinical parameters:
Overall survival (OS)
Progression free-survival (PFS)
Tumor imaging (RECIST)
Tumor metabolism (PET)
Biomarkers:
Tumor-associated antigens (CEA, PSA, CA125, CA19-1,....)
Circulating tumor cells (CTCs)
Release of intracellular antigens during apoptosis/necrosis
Circulating nucleic acids (nDNA, mRNA, miRNA,..)
Intracellular antigens (CKs, CA125, HMGB1, S100B,...)

Table 1. Methods for the assessment of tumor response

2.2.2 Circulating tumor cells

Circulating tumor cells (CTCs) can be released from the primary tumor into the bloodstream and may colonize distant organs giving rise to metastasis (Alunni-Fabbroni & Sandri, 2010). The presence of CTCs in the blood has been documented more than a century ago, and in the meanwhile various methods have been described for their detection and automated enumeration. Most of them require an initial enrichment step, since CTCs are a very rare event. CTCs can be detected in the blood of many patients with different types of early or advanced cancer using antibody-based assays or molecular methods (Mavroudis, 2010).

In many studies the detection and quantification of CTCs has been linked to unfavourable prognosis and CTC detection offers the opportunity for individualized risk assessment superior to TNM staging. However, discordant results have been reported when different methodologies for CTC detection were used (Pantel & Alix-Panabières, 2010). Therefore, well-standardized detection methods cross-validated between different laboratories are still needed. CTCs are a heterogeneous population of cells with biological characteristics often different from those of their respective primary tumor cells. CTCs have been reported to have high apoptotic indices. Pilot studies have shown that phenotyping of CTCs could be used to predict response to targeted therapies. In the era of biological therapeutics, CTC characterization at different time points during the course of disease may provide useful predictive information for the selection of the most appropriate treatment.

2.2.3 Circulating nucleic acids

DNA, mRNA and microRNA are released and circulate in the blood of cancer patients (Schwarzenbach et al., 2011). Since circulating cell-free nucleic acids (cfNAs) in cancer patients often bears similar genetic and epigenetic features to the related tumor DNA, there is evidence that some of the this genetic material originates from tumoral tissue. Changes in the levels of circulating nucleic acids have been associated with tumor burden and malignant progression. The cfNAs might be excellent blood cancer biomarkers, as they may be more informative, specific and accurate than protein biomarkers. However, to validate the actual clinical application of various cfDNA alterations as potential cancer biomarkers in practice for individual tumor types standardization of the described methods would be a prerequisite.

3. Circulating CKs and CK fragments as tumor biomarkers

3.1 Detection of CK expression in the diagnosis of tumors

Keratins have been recognized as tumor markers in the diagnosis of cancer for over 20 years (Weber et al., 1984; Sundstrom & Stigbrand, 1994). CKs are a family of more than 20 intermediate filament (IF) proteins expressed in cells of epithelial origin and endothelial cells (Ekman et al., 2007; Karantza, 2011). They are subdivided into two groups: CKs 1-8, the type II group comprising neutral to basic proteins of 53-68 kD and CKs 9–20, the type I group including acidic proteins of 40-56 kDa. CKs are composed of complexes of one type I and one type II CK protein that become organized into larger filamentous polymeric structures. The most abundant CKs are 8, 18 and 19, and a common example of the heteropolymer complex is the combination of CKs 8 and 18. Commonly, the tissue-specific CK expression profile is stable, even during malignant transformation and, therefore, it is utilized in pathology to distinguish different tumor entities. CK8, CK18 and CK19 are expressed by most types of carcinomas, including those of the breast, prostate, lung, colon and ovary. Under normal physiological conditions CKs are complexed in IF of epithelial cells and remain insoluble (Fuchs & Weber, 1994). Proliferating cancer cells also contain a substantial pool of soluble CKs (CK8, 18 and 19), which can increase in response to stress (Schutte et al., 2004). In the circulation CKs are present as large or small protein complexes or in form of partially degraded single-protein fragments (Ku et al., 1997). The levels of circulating CKs are significantly increased in patients with epithelia-derived malignancies (Linder, 2007). The exact mechanism of the release of the CKs may involve release of intact proteins from rapidly proliferating tumor cells or cell death (Linder et al., 2004). Most type I CKs display caspase cleavage sites allowing for the detection of apoptotic cell death through assessment of newly formed epitopes in the process of their specific degradation. During necrosis, mobilization of CK18 into the soluble pool occurs through remodelling of the IFs (Strnad et al., 2002), whereas during apoptosis IF proteins (including CK18) are targeted for rapid breakdown by activated caspases 3, 7 and 9 to facilitate the formation of apoptotic bodies (Kramer et al., 2004). Several monoclonal anti-CK antibodies are available that recognize the most abundant CKs, i.e. 8, 18 and 19 (Stigbrand et al., 1998). The three most commonly applied CK markers overall are TPA, TPS and CYFRA 21-1. TPA is a broad-spectrum test that measures CKs 8, 18 and 19, while TPS and CYFRA 21-1 measure CKs 18 and 19, respectively (Weber et al., 1984; Stieber et al., 1993; Sundström et al., 1994; Stigbrand et al., 1998; Barak et al., 2004).

M30® and M65® (Peviva AB, Bromma, Sweden) are sandwich ELISA assays that determine different circulating forms of the CK18 in either plasma or serum and are proposed to be surrogate biomarkers of different mechanisms of cell death (Biven et al., 2003; Kramer et al., 2004). The M30 ELISA assay utilizes the M5 anti-CK antibody as a catcher and the M30 antibody to detect CK18 fragments that contain a neoepitope at positions 387–396 generated by the action of caspases 3, 7 and 9 activated during the early stages of apoptosis (Leers et al., 1999; Schutte et al., 2004). CK18 fragments detected by the M30 Apoptosense assay are frequently referred to as "M30" in the literature, which is incorrect since M30 is an antibody and not an antigen (Linder, 2011). The fragments can be referred to as "ccCK18" (caspase-cleaved CK18). Alternatively, since there is a second caspase-cleavage site in the CK18 molecule at Asp237, a more precise terminology would be "K18Asp396".

Thus, the M30 ELISA is proposed as a specific assay for apoptosis and immunological staining with the M30 (Cytodeath®) antibody has been shown to correlate with other apoptosis assays such as terminal deoxynucleotidyl transferase dUTP nick end labeling (TUNEL) and presence of active caspase 3 (Carr, 2000; Duan et al., 2003). M65 also detects cleaved fragments; however, it uses a different detection antibody from M30 (namely M5) that does not distinguish between the full-length protein and its fragments (Kramer et al., 2004). Thus, M65 theoretically measures both caspase cleavage (apoptosis) and cellular release of intact CK18 (necrosis). None of the cell types that normally circulate in blood express CK18, neither do dividing and chemotherapy-sensitive cells of the bone marrow. Carcinoma cells may also contain fragmented CK molecules, presumably owing to increased levels of proteolytic enzymes in the cytosol of tumor cells. The CK18 material present in the circulation of cancer patients consists of higher-molecular-weight complexes between different types of CKs. In addition to such complexes, cells release shorter polypeptide fragments that have short half-lifes in the circulation and are not detected in patient serum (Linder, 2010). It is an advantage that CKs are present as complexes in the circulation, since such aggregates are relatively stable during storage of serum/plasma and survive multiple freeze–thawing cycles.

Both M30 and M65 assays have now been applied extensively in clinical trials as biomarkers of cell death induced by a variety of different cancer chemotherapeutic agents in a spectrum of different disease types (Biven et al., 2003; Ueno et al., 2003; Kramer et al., 2004, 2006; Demiray et al., 2006; Ulukaya et al., 2007). In some preliminary reports, the M30 assay has been claimed to be both predictive of drug response (Demiray et al., 2006) and prognostic of survival (Ulukaya et al., 2007). The two ELISAs have also been utilized as markers of host tissue toxicity in a number of different clinical conditions including trauma, sepsis (Roth et al., 2004), chronic liver disease (Yagmur et al., 2007), hepatitis C (Bantel et al., 2004) and in liver transplantation (Baskin-Bey et al., 2007).

3.2 CKs and tumor cell death

Within the era of molecularly targeted anticancer agents it has become increasingly important to provide proof of mechanism as early as possible. Selective activation of apoptosis is one of the major goals of cancer chemotherapy (Kepp et al., 2011). Serological assays utilising ELISA for detection of apoptotic events would have the advantage of sampling multiple time points. Potential biomarkers of apoptosis including CTCs, CKs and nuclear DNA (nDNA) are discussed at length (Ward et al., 2008). However, accepting that a single biomarker may not have the power to predict proof of concept and patient outcome and technologies that can analyse panels of biomarkers in small volumes of samples will be a future necessity.

A hallmark of neoplasia is dysregulated apoptosis or programmed cell death (Hotchkiss et al., 2009). Dysregulation of apoptotic pathways leads to reduced responses to chemotherapeutic drugs or radiation and is a frequent contributor to therapeutic resistance in cancer. Virtually all methods for detecting apoptosis, including classic cytomorphologic evaluation, TUNEL assay, immunocytochemistry, and gene sequence analysis, may be applied to cytologic samples as well as tissue (Shtilbans et al., 2010). Early morphological features of apoptosis include blebbing of the cell surface, after which cell shrinkage, cytoskeletal rearrangements, chromatin condensation, and nuclear fragmentation occur. The duration of the apoptotic process is about 12–24 hours. As cells proceed to apoptosis, phosphatidylserine (PS), a lipid normally facing the cytoplasm, flips and faces the extracellular fluid. The protein annexin V binds PS strongly, specifically in a calcium-dependent fashion, which is a reflection of its biologic role as an anticoagulant. Attempts to image apoptotic tumor cells with help of fluorescent active Cy-annexin V and surface reflectance fluorescence to determine chemosensitivity were performed successfully in xenografts; however, clinical application is under development (Schellenberger et al., 2003). In addition to the reduced trauma to patients compared to obtaining surgical samples, the use of repeat cytologic sampling before and after cancer therapy to monitor therapy-induced apoptosis and rapidly predict therapeutic response, shows promise in several studies and may become increasingly valuable as cancer therapy becomes more individualized, based upon drug responsiveness of each individual patient's tumor. Thus, apoptotic products released into blood circulation are suggested as promising markers for the early cancer detection (Holdenrieder & Stieber, 2004, 2010). However, though sensitive assays are available, the lack of organ- and tumor-specificity limits the usefulness of most apoptotic parameters for screening purposes. Nevertheless, they seem to be valuable for the prognosis and the prediction of response to systemic chemo- or radiotherapy in cancer disease. Among those promising markers are ligands and receptors of the FAS-system, members of the intracellular caspase cascade, cleaved apoptosis substrates such as CK fragments, nDNA and apoptosis modulators like survivin.

3.3 Levels of circulating CKs and fragments in tumor patients

A number of groups have demonstrated elevated levels of CK18 and/or ccCK18 in serum/plasma from patients with various forms of carcinomas, including breast (Ueno et al., 2003; Demiray et al., 2006), colon (Koelink et al., 2009; Ausch et al., 2009a,b), lung (Hou et al., 2009; Ulukaya et al., 2007), prostate (Kramer et al., 2004, 2006), testicular (de Haas et al., 2008), head and neck (Ozturk et al., 2009), pancreatic (Dive et al., 2010) and gastrointestinal adenocarcinoma (Scott et al., 2009; Yaman et al., 2010). Increases of baseline ccCK18 were believed to mirror spontaneous apoptosis of tumor cells and appeared to be of clinical significance. Increased circulating amounts of ccCK18 were reported to be associated to the number of involved organs, performance status and shorter median survival (Ueno et al., 2003; Koelink et al., 2009; Ulukaya et al., 2007).

The potential diagnostic and prognostic significance of circulating CK18 and ccCK18 was investigated in patients with non-small-cell lung cancer (NSCLC) in comparison with CYFRA 21.1, a fragment of cytokeratin 19 (De Petris et al., 2011). Subject cohorts consisted of

200 healthy blood donors, 113 patients with benign lung diseases and 179 NSCLC cases. Plasma levels of both ccCK18 and total CK18 were higher in the NSCLC group compared to the healthy controls and the cohort with benign diseases. The diagnostic accuracy of both CK18 forms to distinguish between NSCLC and nonmalignant control cases was 56%, whereas it was 94% for CYFRA 21.1. Multivariate survival analysis showed that total CK18 was a stronger prognostic factor than both ccCK18 and CYFRA 21.1., while ccCK18 was not of prognostic value, suggesting that tumor necrosis is of particular importance in this disease. Two studies were published evaluating CK18 in patients with colorectal cancer. The first studied pre- and postoperative serum levels of ccCK18 in 31 patients (Ausch et al., 2009b). Persisting levels of ccCK18 after apparently radical surgery on colon cancer patients correlated significantly with disease recurrence. The second study measured pre- and postoperative plasma levels of ccCK18 and total CK18 in 49 patients with colorectal cancer and correlated the levels with patient and tumor characteristics as well as OS (Koelink et al., 2009). The results showed that perioperative plasma levels of both ccCK18 and total CK18 were correlated with disease stage and were predictive of DFS independent of tumor stage. However, in none of these reports the determination of circulating CK18 reached sufficient accuracy to be proposed as a potential diagnostic assay. A positive predictive correlation between baseline circulating CK18 levels and patient outcome has been suggested in several other tumor diseases such as gastrointestinal adenocarcinomas (Brandt et al., 2010), testis tumors (de Haas et al., 2008), lung cancer (Hou et al., 2009; Ulukaya et al., 2007) and pancreatic cancer (Dive et al., 2010). In general, high pretreatment CK18 levels indicated a larger tumor burden and a less favourable prognosis.

An obvious concern in respect to the use of CK18 as a tumor biomarker is whether circulating CK18 is released from tumor and not from other cells. A number of observations from various studies suggested that CKs are indeed shed by tumor cells. For example, in patients with endometrial carcinoma, CK18 levels were higher in local tumor veins compared with peripheral blood in the same patients (Kramer et al., 2004) and CK18 levels generally decreased after surgical removal of tumors (Ausch et al., 2009a). It is, therefore, very likely that increased baseline levels of CK18 in patients serum/plasma is due to release by the tumor. Caspase activity has been detected in circulation in patients with malignancies (Linder et al., 2010). Therefore, a concern in the analysis of caspase-cleaved fragment in blood as a measure of cellular apoptosis is that cleavage of CK18 might occur in the circulation. Incubation of CK18-positive serum samples with 1,000 units/mL recombinant caspase-3 for 4 hours did not increase the levels of ccCK18 fragments. The association between CK18 markers and the number of CTCs observed by Hou et al. in patients treated with platinum-based therapy seems to provide another strong indication that plasma CK18 originates from the tumor (Hou et al., 2009). Furthermore, the association between CK18 increases and tumor response or patient outcome observed in various studies suggested that CK18 is derived from tumor cells disintegrated in response to cytotoxic therapy. It can, however, not be excluded that increased levels of circulating CK18 are due to higher degrees of drug exposure and may reflect higher toxicity (e.g., to liver tissue).

An expected relationship between plasma CK18 levels and signs of cell death was investigated using tumor histopathology slides of resected pancreatic cancers (Dive et al., 2010). On microscopic assessment one third of the patients exhibited significant areas of tumor necrosis (i.e. > 5%) but without any correlation with plasma M65 levels. Furthermore approximately half of the available cases showed positive staining for activated caspase-3, again without any significant relation to the median plasma ccCK18/M65 ratio between positive and negative cases. This finding seems to implicate that additional factors other than intrinsic tumor biology have an important interfering effect on circulating M65 concentrations. Hepatocytes express CK18 and cancer therapeutics that induced liver toxicity may have evoked release of CK18. A marked correlation was seen between the concurrent bilirubin levels of the pancreatic cancer patients and circulating CK18 levels pointing to obstruction of the main bile duct as cause of cell death within the biliary epithelium and release of CKs in good accordance with findings in cholangitis and chronic liver disease (Yagmur et al., 2007). Endothelial cells, kidney and colon epithelia may shed CK18 and fragments in response to damaging agents due to side effects on normal tissues. Whether CK biomarkers are sufficiently specific for the assessment of apoptosis and necrosis of carcinoma cells to be useful for treatment decisions in routine clinical care is questionable.

3.4 Changes of circulating CK18 and ccCK18 in response to chemotherapeutic drugs

In regard to the potential use of CK18 as a serum biomarker for monitoring therapy efficacy in carcinoma patients supportive data have been reported by different investigators (Linder et al., 2010). A number of groups have observed increased levels of ccCK18 (M30) and/or CK18 (M65) in serum/plasma during cytotoxic therapy of cancer patients (Hou et al., 2009; Kramer et al., 2004; Demiray et al., 2006; Kramer et al., 2006, de Haas et al., 2008; Olofsson et al., 2007). Preclinical results in animal experimental studies discussed in the following raised the hope of successful validitation of these assays in clinical practise.

3.4.1 Animal experimental studies of CK18 fragments of tumor xenografts

Drug-induced increases of ccCK18/CK18 were observed in animal studies using human xenograft tumors (Olofsson et al., 2009; Cummings et al., 2008; Micha et al., 2008). Such increases are certain to originate from tumor cells, since the M30 and M5 antibodies utilized in the M30-Apoptosense and M65 assays detect human but not murine CK18 (Linder et al., 2010). The kinetics of increases in plasma ccCK18 was paralleled by increases in apoptosis in tumor tissue. The M30-Apoptosense therefore permits the specific determination of drug-induced apoptosis in human tumor xenografts in rodents using plasma samples, largely independently from host toxicity.

In detail, treatment of nontumor-bearing rats with the aurora kinase inhibitor AZD1152 produced no alterations in circulating baseline levels of ccCK18 and CK18 (Cummings et al., 2008). In treated tumor-bearing animals, the M30 and M65 assays detected a 2- to 3-fold increase in plasma ccCK18 but not CK18 levels by day 5 compared with controls. This correlated to a 3-fold increase in the number of apoptotic cells detected at the same time point in SW620 xenografts using immunohistochemistry. However, CK18 plasma levels correlated to changes in tumor growth in control animals. It was concluded that ccCK18 represents a pharmacodynamic biomarker of AZD1152-induced apoptosis in the SW620 xenograft model, whereas circulating CK18 is a biomarker of therapeutic response. Furthermore, cell death of SCLC xenografts in mice was measured with help of circulating CK18 in response to a proapoptotic dose of the BH-3 mimetic ABT-737 (Micha et al., 2008). Circulating CK18 levels correlated with tumor burden and ABT-737 caused apoptotic tumor regression in SCLC H146 xenografts indicated by a drug-specific and early increase in ccCK18 that subsequently declined (2 - 24 hrs and 15 days). In summary, in murine xenograft models, in the absence of interference of cell death of normal epithelial tissues, CK18 and ccCK18 were valid markers of tumor mass and response, respectively.

3.4.2 Cytotoxic chemotherapy and circulating ccCK18 and CK18

As discussed above, the amount of ccCK18 which has accumulated in cells or tissue culture media during apoptosis is measured by the M30-ELISA and the M65-ELISA assay will detect all CK18 species that contain epitopes in the 300 to 390 amino acid region of the protein (Biven et al., 2003). Chemotherapeutic agents commonly induce apoptosis with slow kinetics over 24 hours. For example, cisplatin, etoposide and paclitaxel typically induce CK18 cleavage after more than 12 hours of incubation. During paclitaxel-induced apoptosis of human breast cancer cells, approximately 10^{-5} U of ccCK18 ccCK18 is generated per cell. This means that induction of apoptosis in 10% of the cells of a tumor containing 10^{9} cells will generate approximately 1000 U ccCK18. In a plasma volume of 3 L, this will lead to a concentration of 330 U/L compared to a baseline level of approximately 150 U/L in normal subjects that would be easily detected (Biven et al., 2003). Bone marrow is one of the major organs affected by antineoplastic drugs, but since CK18 is only expressed in epithelial cells, apoptosis in bone marrow will not contribute to increases in M30-reactive material during chemotherapy. Selected studies on circulating CK18 and ccCK18 are listed in table 2.

In a study in 32 patients with recurrent breast cancer receiving chemotherapy with cyclophosphamide, epirubicin and 5-fluorouracil (5-FU) or docetaxel (Biven et al., 2003), an index was calculated for each patient based on the difference between the maximum ccCK18 level observed during treatment and the pretreatment level. Increases by 50% or more were observed in 57% of responders compared to 5.6% of the nonresponders. Release of the cytosolic pool of soluble CK18 during necrotic cell death and of ccCK18 during apoptosis, respectively, was described by Kramer et al. in two studies involving prostate cancer patients (Kramer et al., 2004, 2006). Circulating CKs in patients with hormone refractory prostate cancer receiving palliative chemotherapy showed significant increases in ccCK18, usually between days 5 and 7 of each treatment cycle (Kramer et al, 2006). During sequential treatment with either estramustine/vinorelbine or with estramustine/docetaxel, estramustine alone induced increases in serum CK18, but not in ccCK18, while docetaxel was able to induce significant levels of tumor apoptosis. The magnitude of docetaxel-induced increases in ccCK18 was associated with baseline prostate-specific antigen (PSA) and CK18 serum levels in these patients, providing potential evidence of a tumoral origin of caspase-cleaved fragments. However, toxicity accompanying administration of these combination chemotherapies was not reported. In another study, tumor cell apoptosis and antiapoptotic response was measured by determinations of ccCK18 and soluble Fas (sFas) in serial samples from 42 patients with different cancers under chemotherapy (Pichon et al., 2006). Baseline antiapoptotic sFas was higher in cancer patients than in normal subjects and increased with the number of previous chemotherapy cycles. The median baseline ccCK18 did not differ from normal subjects, but patients with a maximum increase >67.5% during chemotherapy had a better univariate OS. As measured by sFas concentration, chemotherapy induced an anti-apoptotic response of differing intensity according to tumor types and drugs, which had a prognostic value for survival. The effect of four cycles of anthracycline-based neoadjuvant chemotherapy on ccCK18 levels was investigated in a group of 42 patients with invasive breast carcinoma by Demiray et al. and ccCK18 serum concentrations at 24 and 48 hours after initiation of chemotherapy were found to be

AUTHORS	CHEMOTHERAPY	TUMOR ENTITY	# PTS	RESULT(S): CK18/ccCK18
Kramer et al. 2004	Estramustine/ vinorelbine	prostate cancer	25	M65+ upon cell death
Pichon et al. 2006	chemotherapy	epidermoid/ carcinoma	42	+ correlation with survival
Kramer et al. 2006	Estramustine-based	prostate cancer	82	ccCK18+ upon docetaxel therapy
Demiray et al. 2006	Anthracycline-based	breast cancer	42	d1 + d2 peaks in responders
Olofsson et al. 2007	Docetaxel/CEF	breast cancer	61	ccCK18+ in response to docetaxel M65+ in responders on CEF
Steele et al. 2008	Belinostat (HDAC inhibitor)	solid tumors	46	d2 +d8, in responders
de Haas EC et al. 2008	BEP	testicular cancer	34	d7 +, peaks similar in nonresponders
Scott et al. 2009	5-FU/platinum	gastrointestinal cancer	73	M65+ in responders
Hou et al. 2009	platinum/etoposide	SCLC	88	+ apoptotic CTC/ liver toxicity
Lickliter et al. 2010	CYT997 (microtubule inhibitor)	solid tumors/Phase 1	31	d1+, dose-dependent increase
Le Tourneau et al. 2010	Seleciclib (CDK inhibitor)	advanced tumor/Phase 1	56	+ dose-dependent increase + metastatic patients and toxicity d2
Brandt et al. 2010	5-FU/combination	gastrointestinal cancer	35	cycle end, ccCK18+ in responders
Ulukaya et al. 2011	FEC/ED	breast cancer	37	d1+d2, increase (also in 1 nonresponder)
Shin et al. 2011	TSU-68 (TK inhibitor) + S-1/oxaliplatin	mCRC/Phase 1	11	no significant changes upon therapy
Mahadevan et al. 2011	AT7519 (CDK inhibitor)	solid tumors/Phase 1	28	d5+, correlated with tumor apoptosis
Greystoke et al. 2011	ABVD/R-CVP/R-CHOP	lymphoma	49	d3+, correlated with epithelial toxicity
Gandhi et al. 2011	Navitoclax (Bcl2 inhibitor)	SCLC/carcinoid/ others	47	transient peak after 6 hrs
Dean et al. 2011	Obatoclax + carbo-platin/etoposide	SCLC Phase 1b-2	24	no ccCK18+ with Bcl2 inhibitor

Table 2. Overview of studies dealing with measurements of CK18 and/or ccCK18 in patients receiving conventional or targeted chemotherapy.

significantly higher than baseline in responders, while such increases were not observed in nonresponders (Demiray et al., 2006). Docetaxel induced increased levels of ccCK18 in serum from breast cancer patients, indicating apoptosis (Olofsson et al., 2007). Neoadjuvant cyclophosphamide/ epirubicin/ 5-fluorouracil (CEF) therapy led to increases predominantly in uncleaved CK18, indicating necrotic cell death. The increase in total CK18 at 24 h of the first treatment cycle correlated to the clinical response to CEF therapy.

Disseminated testicular germ cell cancer (TC) is a paradigm for a solid malignancy of epithelial origin chemosensitive to bleomycin/ etoposide/ cisplatin (BEP). The peaks of CK18 and ccCK18 observed after the start of each treatment cycle in good and intermediate-prognosis group patients indicated a drug-induced effect, which may have reflected tumor response (de Haas et al., 2008). However, the fact that these peaks are not observed in patients with poor prognosis was possibly related to high initial levels of CK18 and ccCK18. With this analysis in a small number of selected patients it could not be proven that CK18 and ccCk18 peaks were specific enough to prove chemotherapy-induced tumor cell death. Neither could it be excluded that these peaks (partially) reflected chemotherapy-induced toxicity to normal epithelial tissues. The four patients with TC who eventually did not respond to BEP chemotherapy after an initial decline in tumor markers showed patterns of circulating CK18 and ccCK18 comparable to responding patients. In case these peaks were tumor cell death-related they were interpreted as signs disintegration of chemotherapy-sensitive subpopulations of cells. Consequently, the presence of chemotherapy-induced peaks in CK18 and ccCK18 might not exclude future treatment failure.

Soluble plasma ccCK18 and CK18 were measured from 73 patients and 100 healthy volunteers with advanced gastrointestinal adenocarcinomas before treatment and during chemotherapy (Scott et al., 2009). The majority of the patients with gastric or oesophageal adenocarcinoma were treated with combination chemotherapy comprising epirubicin, cisplatin, and 5-FU and few patients with either cisplatin/5-FU or carboplatin/5-FU. CRC patients were treated with capecitabine monotherapy or in a few cases with 5-FU and folinic acid. Both ccCK18 and total CK18 plasma levels were significantly higher in patients compared with the healthy volunteers. The total CK18 baseline plasma levels before treatment were significantly higher in patients who developed progressive disease and the peak plasma levels of CK18 occurring in any cycle following treatment were also found to be associated with tumor response, but peak levels of ccCK18 did not reach significance. There was an overall sensitivity of 22% at a specificity of 90% for ccCK18 and an overall sensitivity of 19% at a specificity of 90% for CK18 baseline plasma levels in distinguishing between patients who subsequently progressed and those who had partial response/stable disease. Pooled data for all 73 patients demonstrated that ccCK18 has a sensitivity of 27% at a specificity of 90% and CK18 a sensitivity of 71% at a specificity of 90% in distinguishing patients with malignancy and healthy volunteers, respectively. Both markers may have limited use as a diagnostic marker. In the healthy volunteers both plasma ccCK18 and CK18 varied over a wide range. Alcohol intake is known to increase ccCK18 values in serum due to apoptosis of liver cells (Natori et al, 2001). Other studies have also shown that viral illness, chronic hepatitis, and sepsis will increase levels of ccCK18 detected by the M30 Apoptosense ELISA kit (Scott et al., 2009). Hou et al. compared measurements CK18 products in blood samples from 88 SCLC patients with levels of nDNA and numbers of CTCs (Hou et al., 2009). Before treatment, CK18 fragments were elevated in patients compared with controls and ccCK18 levels correlated with the percentage of apoptotic

CTCs. CTC number fell following chemotherapy with cisplatin/etoposide, whereas levels of serological cell death biomarkers peaked at 48 hours and fell by day 22, mirroring tumor response. A 48-hour rise in nDNA and ccCK18 levels was associated with early response and severe toxicity, respectively. Levels of nDNA did not correlate with M65 or ccCK18. Persistently elevated ccCk18 and CTC number at day 22 were adverse prognostic factors in univariate analysis. There was a significant association between an increase in nDNA at 48 hours and response compared with stable disease. Patients who developed toxicity requiring hospitalization had higher baseline levels of cell death biomarkers, potentially reflecting a higher disease burden and poorer performance status before therapy. The peak in ccCK18 at 48 hours was significantly higher in patients requiring admission for toxicity.

The putative association of serum CK-18 levels and clinical response was furthermore investigated in 35 patients with gastrointestinal cancers (Brandt et al., 2010). While both cleaved and total CK-18 levels were intrinsically elevated in tumor patients, they were further increased during 5-FU-based therapy. Cancer patients with a partial response or stable disease revealed a significantly higher increase of ccCK-18 during chemotherapy as compared to patients with progressive disease. Our own group assessed serum levels of ccCK18 in 10 CRC patients receiving combination chemotherapy with oxaliplatin/capecitabine and observed that increases in ccCK18 during chemotherapy did not correlate with tumor response (Ausch et al, 2009a). A breast cancer study of CK18 was perfomed by Ulukaya et al. employing 37 patients as well as 35 patients with benign breast disease and 34 healthy subjects for comparison (Ulukaya et al., 2011). Cancer patients received neoadjuvant chemotherapy consisting of either 5-FU, epirubicin, and cyclophosphamide (FEC) or epirubicin plus docetaxel (ED). Apoptosis was assessed before chemotherapy and 24 and 48 h after chemotherapy in the malignant group. It was found that the baseline apoptosis levels in either nonmetastatic malignant or benign group were not statistically different from that in the control group, but elevated in the metastatic cancer group. Following drug application, ccCK18 levels significantly increased about 3-fold in patients showing tumor regression at 24 h but not in nonresponders. However, the single progressive patient revealed an almost 5-fold increase in ccCK18. It is possible that these findings can be explained by therapeutic response, showing a stronger correlation to total cell death (apoptosis and necrosis) compared with apoptosis alone. Indeed, whether cytotoxic drugs kill tumor cells *in vivo* by apoptosis or necrosis is controversial (Kaufmann & Vaux, 2003; Zong & Thompson, 2006).

Circulating biomarkers of cell death such as nDNA, CK18 and circulating FLT3 ligand, a potential biomarker of myelosuppression, were assessed before and serially after standard chemotherapy in 49 patients with Hodgkin and non-Hodgkin lymphoma (Greystoke et al., 2011). CK18 is not expressed in lymphoma cells and thus represented a potential biomarker of epithelial toxicity in this setting. Decreases in nDNA levels were observed in the first week after chemotherapy; Circulating CK18 increased within 48 hours of chemotherapy and was significantly higher in patients experiencing epithelial toxicity graded >3 by Common Terminology for Classification of Adverse Events criteria (CTCAE).

3.4.3 Targeted chemotherapy and changes in circulating CK18 and ccCK18

Determinations of ccCK18 may also be applicable as a pharmacodynamic biomarker in phase I clinical trials of novel noncytotoxic molecularly targeted anticancer therapies, with which objective tumor responses, as determined by a reduction in tumor dimensions by conventional imaging techniques, may not be observed. Several groups reported measurements of CK18 and CK18 fragments in clinical studies of such agents.

CYT997 is a novel microtubule inhibitor and vascular-disrupting agent with marked preclinical antitumor activity (Lickliter et al., 2010). Moreover, plasma levels of von Willebrand factor and ccC18 increased post-treatment at higher dose levels. Among 22 patients evaluable for response, 18 achieved stable disease for >2 cycles. Seventeen patients in this study were evaluable for the analysis of ccCK18 levels, which were observed to increase at 24 h after commencing CYT997 in a dose-dependent manner. In another study, 56 patients received a total of 218 cycles of the cyclin-dependent kinase (CDK) inhibitor seliciclib (Le Tourneau et al., 2010). Soluble CK18 fragments allowed detection of seliciclib-induced cell death in the blood of patients treated at doses above 800 mg/day. Another CDK inhibitor, namely AT7519, afforded stable disease for >6 months in four out of 28 patients and a prolonged partial response in one patient bearing solid tumors (Mahadevan et al., 2011). Inhibition of markers of CDK activity was observed across the dose range and manifested in antiproliferative activity. A consistent decrease in Ki67 levels and increase in both the cleaved and intact forms of CKs were observed in the majority of samples, suggesting that AT7519 was inducing tumor cell apoptosis.

Disease stabilisation was associated with ccCK18 plasma levels in patients with advanced solid tumors treated in a phase 1 clinical trial of the novel hydroxamate histone deacetylase (HDAC) inhibitor, belinostat (Steele et al, 2008). Of the 24 patients treated at the maximum tolerated dose, 50% achieved stable disease and ccCK18 levels were significantly increased on days 2 and 8 in patients with stable disease but showed no significant elevation in patients with progressive disease. Consistent with this epitope being derived from tumor and not normal cells undergoing therapy-induced apoptosis, patients who did not have epithelial cancer showed no change in level of ccCK18 during treatment. No significant mean changes of ccCK18 after administration of each of several cycles of chemotherapy was observed in a phase I study evaluating the safety and pharmacokinetic of TSU-68, when used with S-1 (combination of tegafur, gimeracil and oteracil) and oxaliplatin (SOX) in mCRC patients (Shin et al., 2011). TSU-68 is a novel multiple tyrosine kinase inhibitor that inhibits VEGFR-2, FGF and PDGF receptors.

SCLC is an aggressive disease in which, after initial sensitivity to platinum/etoposide chemotherapy, patients frequently relapse with drug-resistant disease. Deregulation of the Bcl-2 pathway is implicated in the pathogenesis of SCLC, and early phase studies of Bcl-2 inhibitors were initiated in SCLC. A phase I study of navitoclax, a novel inhibitor of Bcl-2 family proteins, was conducted (Gandhi et al., 2011). Forty-seven patients, including 29 with SCLC or pulmonary carcinoid, were enrolled. A dose-dependent transient increase after 6 hours in circulating ccCK18 was observed in higher dose cohorts. Obatoclax represents another small-molecule drug designed to target the antiapoptotic Bcl-2 family members to a proapoptotic effect (Dean et al., 2011). In vitro, obatoclax was synergistic with cisplatin and etoposide, and priming of cells with obatoclax before the cytotoxics maximized tumor cell death. Peak levels of apoptosis, reflected by ccCK18 levels and caspase activity, occurred 24 hours after obatoclax treatment. A phase 1b-2 trial of obatoclax administered using two infusion regimens in combination with carboplatin and etoposide was completed in previously untreated patients with extensive-stage SCLC. All SCLC patients classified as responders after two cycles of treatment showed significantly increased levels of full-length and cleaved CK18 on day 3 of the study. However, in difference to the preclinical data a peak in circulating ccCK18 was not detectable in trial patients and explained by a suboptimal timing of blood sampling.

Dulanermin (rhApo2L/TRAIL) induces apoptosis by binding to death receptors DR4 and DR5, leading to caspase activation and subsequent cell death (Pan et al., 2011). A preclinical study using Colo205 xenografts revealed a transient increase of ccCK18 in response to dulanermin that peaked around 24 hours and gradually declined thereafter. A Phase 1a trial evaluated the safety and tolerability of dulanermin in patients with advanced tumors. In two out of seven NSCLC patients with evaluable biomarker measurements at baseline, a significant increase of cell-death biomarkers was observed 5 hours after dulanermin administration. In CRC patients increases in cleaved CK18 at 24 hours post dulanermin treatment relative to baseline were also observed. Circulating caspase 3/7 increased in a statistically significant manner in CRC and sarcoma patients treated with dulanermin. Remarkably, in contrast to the preclinical results, the clinical analysis showed little correlation between cell-death markers and tumor response.

4. Acute side effects of chemotherapy and relation to tumor response

Chemotherapeutic drugs act on rapidly multiplying tumor and normal cells accounting for both response and the toxic side effects. Therefore, a significant correlation may exist between the effects of the agents and the toxicity produced. The time course of various toxicities depends on the drug, its dose and frequency of administration, intrinsic characteristics of the affected tissue of interest and other factors. Mucosal toxicities of pain, erythema, ulceration etc. occur 3–10 days after the administration of respective drugs and bone marrow effects are detectable between days 7–14 after initiation of treatment. The recovery of normal cellular function is ongoing 4–5 days after culmination of these toxic effects. Cytotoxic drugs, in particular 5-FU, impair replacement of intestinal epithelia and induce flattening of the villi, leading to increased exposure of luminal contents to crypts and increased absorption (Melichar & Zezulova, 2011). Intestinal permeability changes correlated with clinical manifestations, including diarrhea, mucositis, neutropenic enterocolitis and systemic infections. After chemotherapy apoptosis increased sevenfold in intestinal crypts at one day, and villus area, crypt length, mitotic count per crypt, and enterocyte height decreased at three days followed by recovery after 16 days (Keefe et al., 2000).

Several studies reported correlations between toxic side effects and tumor responses induced by chemotherapeutic drugs. Dahl et al. described a correlation between an adverse reaction of normal bowel and radiation sensitivity of presumably operable rectal adenocarcinomas derived from the same tissue (Dahl et al., 1994). Patients experiencing severe side effects including necessary medication had significantly smaller tumors at subsequent surgery. These patients had less recurrence and better disease-specific survival rates than did patients without high-grade acute side effects. In 303 patients with advanced CRC the relationship between chemotherapy-associated adverse events and treatment efficacy was investigated using toxicity, objective response and survival data (Schuell et al., 2005). The results of this study suggested that the frequency of side effects during chemotherapy in advanced CRC was an independent and reliable prognostic indicator for response and survival.

During neoadjuvant chemotherapy for breast cancer responders revealed significant toxicity while nonresponders did not (Chintamani et al., 2004). The chemotherapy-induced toxicity was concluded to be a cost-effective and reliable predictor of response to this type of chemotherapy. The putative association between acute organ toxicity with treatment outcome was investigated in patients with locally advanced head and neck squamous cell carcinoma (HNSCC) during adjuvant radiation and chemotherapy (Wolff et al., 2011). Patients varied in their disposition to side effects during therapy, independently of treatment regimen and high-grade acute organ toxicity during radiation and chemotherapy was associated with better outcomes. Treatment response was variable among patients and tumor types most likely due to individual differences in cellular sensitivity. These data point to a similar behaviour of normal and tumor tissues with respect to treatment response. Finally, Bonner et al. showed that in patients with locally advanced HNSCC treated with radiation therapy and cetuximab, acute toxicity (rash and skin toxicity) could also predict tumor response (Bonner et al., 2010). The correlation of skin rashes with a significantly better OS in lung cancer patients receiving anti-EGF-receptor therapy was reviewed by Perez-Soler (Perez-Soler, 2006).

In conclusion, damage to normal tissues is suggested to be associated with increased tumor response in several carcinomas and for specific chemotherapeutic regimens. Therefore, it cannot be excluded that increases in circulating CK18 and ccCK18 in short-term reaction to chemotherapeutic agents are due to toxic side effects and that the larger release of CKs in responding patients is only indirectly correlated with tumor cell death. Elevations of CK fragments in lymphoma patients with CK-negative hematopoietic tumor cells treated with anthracyclines, alkylating agents and Vinca alkaloids clearly indicated cell death of epithelial normal cells and release due to toxic side effects within 2 days of start of chemotherapy (Greystoke et al., 2011). Thus, an idealized course of CK18 during chemotherapeutic treatment is shown in Figure 1. Patients with carcinomas exhibit elevated circulating CK18 and fragments compared to healthy controls (approximately 150 U/L CK18).

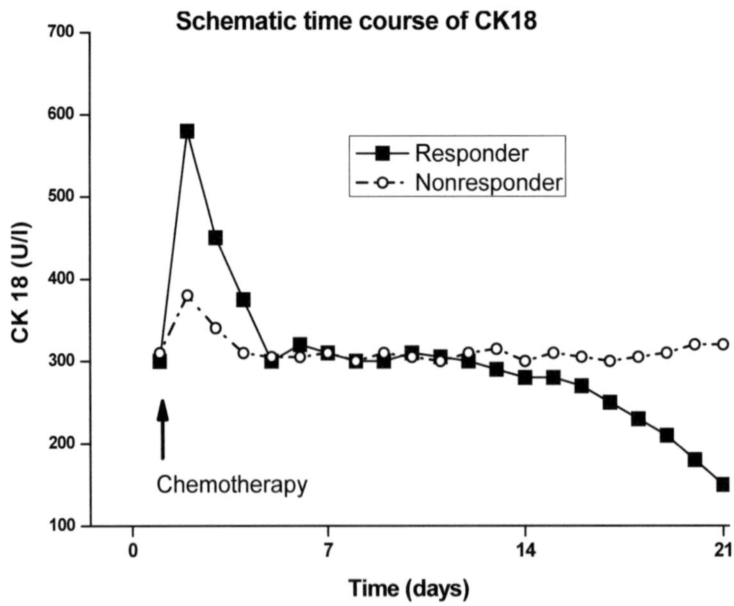

Fig. 1. Schematic course of circulating CK18 typically observed in patients in response to chemotherapy. The two curves summarize results of CK18 in responding and nonresponding patients described in studies shown in table 2.

In responding patients peaks of CK18 within 5 - 48 hours after initiation of treatment are typically observed that seem to coincide with the maximal plasma concentrations of the drugs. The sources of the circulating CKs in this situation seem to be damaged normal tissues like hepatocytes and epithelial cells of the kidney and the gastrointestinal tract as well as tumor cells. In clinical practise, the CK18 assays are not expected to be suitable to discriminate the toxic side effects on normal epithelia and anticancer activity of the drugs. However, residual tumor burden after therapy is indicated by a lack of normalization of circulating CK18 few weeks after start of therapy, well past to the recovery of normal tissues. Nonresponders fail to exhibit drug-induced peaks most likely due to high baseline values of the circulating CKs, that indicate a larger tumor burden, and a possible reduced individual sensitivity to the agents applied.

5. Conclusions

Advances in genomics, proteomics and molecular pathology have generated many candidate biomarkers of potential clinical value (Ludwig & Weinstein, 2005). Their use for cancer staging and personalization of therapy at the time of diagnosis could improve patient care. However, translation from bench to bedside outside of the research setting has proved more difficult than might have been expected. Understanding how and when biomarkers can be integrated into clinical care is crucial if we want to translate the promise into reality. Biomarkers of tumor response to chemotherapy could provide the means to get data on anticancer activity of the agents in preclinical reseach and in clinical setting very rapidly and well in advance of other morphological and clinical data. Released cellular constituents that under normal conditions reside intracellularly could constitute indicators of abnormal cell proliferation or cell death in the peripheral circulation. Different CKs and a caspase-cleaved CK fragments have been employed to detect tumor load, proliferation and tumor necrosis/apoptosis in patients bearing epithelial cancers. While in general a good correlation exists between elevated levels of circulating CK18/ccCK18 and tumor burden of untreated patients, the influence of anticancer treatment with various agents on the release of CKs by tumor cells is less clear. The blood concentration of these CKs has predictive power in various tumor entities since larger tumor have a poorer prognosis in the majority of carcinomas. Measurements of circulating CK18 and ccCK18 before and after chemotherapy using conventional as well as experimental drugs revealed significant increases usually occurring within several hours or a few days within application of the respective agents. Although the levels of these CKs were variable, dependent on tumor entity and drug used, most studies reported higher peak values in responding patients versus nonresponders or those with stable disease. The putative sources of the circulating CK18s are spontaneously dying or drug-damaged tumor cells as well as normal epithelial tissues affected by toxic drug side effects. A study involving lymphoma patients with obviously CK-negative tumor cells demonstrated increased CK levels stemming from toxic effects to normal epithelia in response to chemotherapy and this finding is corroborated by other studies correlating release of CKs with liver toxicity and other severe adverse drug effects. Nevertheless, the positive correlation of increased CK18 levels with clinical response may be partially explained by successful therapeutic intervention in those patients who exhibited more severe toxicity. In summary, the complex mode of the release of CK18s by tumors and normal epithelia in response to various stimuli complicates the interpretation of the results and seems to preclude their use as acute response biomarkers in oncology. However, tumor burden may be assessed by pre- and posttreatment determinations of circulating CK18.

6. References

Alunni-Fabbroni, M. & Sandri, MT. (2010) Circulating tumor cells in clinical practice: Methods of detection and possible characterization. *Methods*, Vol. 50, no. 4, pp. 289-297

Ausch, C., Buxhofer-Ausch, V., Olszewski, U., Schiessel, R., Ogris, E., Hinterberger, W. & Hamilton, G. (2009a) Circulating Cytokeratin 18 Fragment M65-A Potential Marker of Malignancy in Colorectal Cancer Patients. *J Gastrointest Surg.* Vol. 13, no. 11, pp. 2020–2026

Ausch, C., Buxhofer-Ausch, V., Olszewski, U., Hinterberger, W., Ogris, E., Schiessel, R. & Hamilton, G. (2009b) Caspase-cleaved cytokeratin 18 fragment (M30) as marker of postoperative residual tumor load in colon cancer patients. *Eur J Surg Oncol.* Vol. 35, no. 11, pp. 1164–1168

Bantel, H., Lügering, A., Heidemann, J., Volkmann, X., Poremba, C., Strassburg, CP., Manns, MP. & Schulze-Osthoff, K. (2004) Detection of apoptotic caspase activation in sera from patients with chronic HCV infection is associated with fibrotic liver injury. *Hepatology*, Vol. 40, no. 5, pp. 1078-1087

Barak, V., Goike, H., Panaretakis, KW. & Einarsson, R. (2004) Clinical utility of cytokeratins as tumor markers. *Clin Biochem.* Vol. 37, no. 7, pp. 529-540

Baskin-Bey, ES., Washburn, K., Feng, S., Oltersdorf, T., Shapiro, D., Huyghe, M., Burgart, L., Garrity-Park, M., van Vilsteren, FG., Oliver, LK., Rosen, CB. & Gores, GJ. (2007) Clinical Trial of the Pan-Caspase Inhibitor, IDN-6556, in Human Liver Preservation Injury. *Am J Transplant.* Vol. 7, no. 1, 218-225

Beck, EP., Moldenhauer, A., Merkle, E., Kiesewetter, F., Jäger, W., Wildt, L. & Lang, N. (1998) CA 125 production and release by ovarian cancer cells in vitro. *Int J Biol Markers*, Vol. 13, no. 4, pp. 200–206

Bonner, JA., Harari, PM., Giralt, J., Cohen, RB., Jones, CU., Sur, RK., Raben, D., Baselga, J., Spencer, SA., Zhu, J., Youssoufian, H., Rowinsky EK. & Ang, KK. (2010) Radiotherapy plus cetuximab for locoregionally advanced head and neck cancer: 5-year survival data from a phase 3 randomised trial, and relation between cetuximab-induced rash and survival. *Lancet Oncol.* Vol. 11, no. 1, pp. 21-28

Biven, K., Erdal, H., Hägg, M., Ueno, T., Zhou, R., Lynch, M., Rowley, B., Wood, J., Zhang, C., Toi, M., Shoshan, MC. & Linder, S. (2003) A novel assay for discovery and characterization of pro-apoptotic drugs and for monitoring apoptosis in patient sera. *Apoptosis*, Vol. 8, no. 3, pp. 263-268

Brandt, D., Volkmann, X., Anstätt, M., Länger, F., Manns, MP., Schulze-Osthoff, K. & Bantel, H. (2010) Serum biomarkers of cell death for monitoring therapy response of gastrointestinal carcinomas. *Eur J Cancer*, Vol. 46, no. 8, pp. 1464-1473

Candolfi, M., Yagiz, K., Foulad, D., Alzadeh, GE., Tesarfreund, M., Muhammad, AK., Puntel, M., Kroeger, KM., Liu, C., Lee, S., Curtin, JF., King, GD., Lerner, J., Sato, K., Mineharu, Y., Xiong, W., Lowenstein, PR. & Castro, MG. (2009) Release of HMGB1 in response to proapoptotic glioma killing strategies: efficacy and neurotoxicity. *Clin Cancer Res.* Vol. 15, no. 13, pp. 4401-4414

Carden, CP., Sarker, D., Postel-Vinay, S., Yap, TA., Attard, G., Banerji, U., Garrett, MD., Thomas, GV., Workman, P., Kaye, SB. & de Bono, JS. (2010) Can molecular biomarker-based patient selection in Phase I trials accelerate anticancer drug development? *Drug Discov Today*, Vol. 15, no. 3-4, pp. 88-97

Carr, NJ. (2000) M30 expression demonstrates apoptotic cells, correlates with in situ end-labeling, and is associated with Ki-67 expression in large intestinal neoplasms. *Arch Pathol Lab Med*. Vol. 124, no. 12, pp. 1768-1772

Chintamani. S., Singhal, V., Singh, JP., Lyall, A., Saxena, S. & Bansal A. (2004) Is drug-induced toxicity a good predictor of response to neo-adjuvant chemotherapy in patients with breast cancer?--a prospective clinical study. *BMC Cancer*, Vol. 13, no. 4, pp. 48

Cummings, J., Hodgkinson, C., Odedra, R Sini, P., Heaton, SP., Mundt, KE., Ward, TH., Wilkinson, RW., Growcott, J., Hughes, A. & Dive C. (2008b) Preclinical evaluation of M30 and M65 ELISAs as biomarkers of drug induced tumor cell death and antitumor activity. *Mol Cancer Ther*. Vol. 7, no. 3, pp. 455–463

Dahl, O., Horn, A. & Mella, O. (1994) Do acute side-effects during radiotherapy predict tumor response in rectal carcinoma? *Acta Oncol*. Vol. 33, no. 4, pp. 409-413

Dean, EJ., Cummings, J., Roulston, A., Berger, M., Ranson, M., Blackhall, F. & Dive, C. (2011) Optimization of circulating biomarkers of obatoclax-induced cell death in patients with small cell lung cancer. *Neoplasia*, Vol. 13, no. 4, pp. 339-347

Demiray, M., Ulukaya, EE., Arslan, M., Gokgoz, S., Saraydaroglu, O., Ercan, I., Evrensel, T. & Manavoglu, O. (2006) Response to Neoadjuvant Chemotherapy in Breast Cancer Could be Predictable by Measuring a Novel Serum Apoptosis Product, Caspase-Cleaved Cytokeratin 18: A Prospective Pilot Study. *Cancer Invest*. Vol. 24, no. 7, pp. 669-676

Dive, C., Smith, RA., Garner, E., Ward, T., George-Smith, SS., Campbell, F., Greenhalf, W., Ghaneh, P. & Neoptolemos, JP. (2010) Considerations for the use of plasma cytokeratin 18 as a biomarker in pancreatic cancer. *Br J Cancer*, Vol. 102, no. 3, pp. 577-582

Duan, WR., Garner, DS., Williams, SD., Funckes-Shippy, CL., Spath, IS., & Blomme, EA. (2003) Comparison of immunohistochemistry for activated caspase-3 and cleaved cytokeratin 18 with the TUNEL method for quantification of apoptosis in histological sections of PC-3 subcutaneous xenografts. *J Pathol*. Vol. 199, no. 2, pp. 221-228

Ekman, S., Eriksson, P., Bergström, S., Johansson, P., Goike, H., Gullbo, J., Henriksson, R., Larsson, A. & Bergqvist, M. (2007) Clinical value of using serological cytokeratins as therapeutic markers in thoracic malignancies. *Anticancer Res*. Vol. 27, no. 5B, pp. 3545-3553

Fuchs, E. & Weber, K. (1994) Intermediate filaments: structure, dynamics, function, and disease. *Annu Rev Biochem*. Vol. 63, pp. 345-382

Gandhi, L., Camidge, DR., Ribeiro de Oliveira, M., Bonomi, P., Gandara, D., Khaira, D., Hann, CL., McKeegan, EM., Litvinovich, E., Hemken, PM., Dive, C., Enschede, SH., Nolan, C., Chiu, YL., Busman, T., Xiong, H., Krivoshik, AP., Humerickhouse, R., Shapiro, GI. & Rudin, CM. (2011) Phase I study of Navitoclax (ABT-263), a novel Bcl-2 family inhibitor., in patients with small-cell lung cancer and other solid tumors. *J Clin Oncol*. Vol. 29, no. 7, pp. 909-916

Gauley, J. & Pisetsky, DS. (2009) The translocation of HMGB1 during cell activation and cell death. *Autoimmunity*, Vol. 42, no. 4, pp. 299-301

Ghanem, G., Loir, B., Morandini, R. Sales, F., Lienard, D., Eggermont, A., Lejeune, F. & EORTC Melanoma Group. (2001) On the release and half-life of S100B protein in the peripheral blood of melanoma patients. *Int J Cancer,*Vol. 94, no. 4, pp. 586–590

Goodison, S., Sun, Y. & Urquidi, V. (2010) Derivation of cancer diagnostic and prognostic signatures from gene expression data. *Bioanalysis,* Vol. 2, no. 5, pp. 855-862

Greystoke, A., O'Connor, JP., Linton, K., Taylor, MB., Cummings, J., Ward, T., Maders, F., Hughes, A., Ranson, M., Illidge, TM., Radford, J. & Dive, C. (2011) Assessment of circulating biomarkers for potential pharmacodynamic utility in patients with lymphoma. *Br J Cancer,* Vol. 104, no. 4, pp. 719-725

Gwyther, SJ. & Schwartz, LH. (2008) How to assess anti-tumor efficacy by imaging techniques. *Eur J Cancer,* Vol. 44, no. 1, pp. 39-45

de Haas, EC., di Pietro, A., Simpson, KL., Meijer, C., Suurmeijer, AJ., Lancashire, LJ., Cummings, J., de Jong, S., de Vries, EG., Dive C. & Gietema, JA. (2008) Clinical evaluation of M30 and M65 ELISA cell death assays as circulating biomarkers in a drug-sensitive tumor, testicular cancer. *Neoplasia,* Vol. 10, no. 10, pp. 1041-1048

Holdenrieder, S. & Stieber, P. (2004) Apoptotic markers in cancer. *Clin Biochem.* Vol. 37, no. 7, pp. 605-661

Holdenrieder S. & Stieber, P. (2010) Circulating apoptotic markers in the management of non-small cell lung cancer. *Cancer Biomark.* Vol. 6, no. 3-4, pp. 197-210

Hotchkiss, RS., Strasser, A., McDunn, JE. & Swanson, PE. (2009) Cell death. *N Engl J Med.* Vol. 361, no. 16, pp. 1570-1583

Hou, JM., Greystoke, A., Lancashire, L., Cummings, J., Ward, T., Board, R., Amir, E., Hughes, S., Krebs, M., Hughes, A., Ranson, M., Lorigan, P., Dive, C. & Blackhall, FH. (2009) Evaluation of circulating tumor cells and serological cell death biomarkers in small cell lung cancer patients undergoing chemotherapy. *Am J Pathol.* Vol. 175, no. 2, pp. 808-816

Kaufmann, SH. & Vaux, DL. (2003) Alterations in the apoptotic machinery and their potential role in anticancer drug resistance. *Oncogene,* Vol. 22, no. 47, pp. 7414–7430

Karantza V. (2011) Keratins in health and cancer: more than mere epithelial cell markers. *Oncogene,* Vol. 13, no. 30, pp. 127-138.

Keefe, DM., Brealey, J., Goland, GJ. & Cummins, AG. (2000) Chemotherapy for cancer causes apoptosis that precedes hypoplasia in crypts of the small intestine in humans. *Gut,* Vol. 47, no. 5, pp. 632-637

Kepp, O., Galluzzi, L., Lipinski, M., Yuan, J. & Kroemer G. (2011) Cell death assays for drug discovery. *Nat Rev Drug Discov.* Vol. 10, no. 3, pp. 221-237

Koelink, PJ., Lamers, CB., Hommes, DW. & Verspaget, HW. (2009) Circulating cell death products predict clinical outcome of colorectal cancer patients. BMC Cancer Vol. 9, 88.

Kramer, G., Schwartz, S., Hägg, M., Havelka., A. & Linder, S. (2006) Docetaxel induces apoptosis in hormone refractory prostate carcinomas during multiple treatment cycles. *Br J Cancer,* Vol. 94, no. 11, pp. 1592-1598

Kramer, G., Erdal, H., Mertens, HJ., Nap, M., Mauermann, J., Steiner, G., Marberger, M., Bivén, K., Shoshan, MC. & Linder, S. (2004) Differentiation between cell death modes using measurements of different soluble forms of extracellular cytokeratin 18. *Cancer Res.* Vol. 64, no. 5, pp. 1751-1756

Kroemer, G., Dallaporta, B. & Resche-Rigon, M. (1998) The mitochondrial death/life regulator in apoptosis and necrosis. *Annu Rev Physiol*. Vol. 60, pp. 619-642

Ku, NO., Liao, J. & Omary MB. (1997) Apoptosis generates stable fragments of human type I keratins. *J Biol Chem*. Vol. 272, no. 52, pp. 33197-33203

Leers, MP., Kölgen, W., Björklund, V., Bergman, T., Tribbick, G., Persson, B., Björklund, P., Ramaekers, FC., Björklund, B., Nap, M., Jörnvall, H. & Schutte, B. (1999) Immunocytochemical detection and mapping of a cytokeratin 18 neo-epitope exposed during early apoptosis. *J Pathol*. Vol. 187, no. 5, pp. 567-572

Lickliter, JD., Francesconi, AB., Smith, G., Burge, M., Coulthard, A., Rose, S., Griffin, M., Milne, R., McCarron, J., Yeadon, T., Wilks, A., Cubitt, A., Wyld, DK. & Vasey, PA (2010) Phase I trial of CYT997, a novel cytotoxic and vascular-disrupting agent. *Br J Cancer*, Vol. 103, no. 5, pp. 597-606

Linder, S., Havelka, AM., Ueno, T. & Shoshan, MC. (2004) Determining tumor apoptosis and necrosis in patient serum using cytokeratin 18 as a biomarker. *Cancer Lett*. Vol. 214, no. 1, pp. 1-9

Linder, S., Olofsson, MH., Herrmann, R. & Ulukaya, E. (2010) Utilization of cytokeratin-based biomarkers for pharmacodynamic studies. *Expert Rev Mol Diagn*. Vol. 10, no. 3, pp. 353-359

Linder, S. (2011) Caspase-cleaved keratin 18 as a biomarker for non-alcoholic steatohepatitis (NASH) - The need for correct terminology. *J Hepatol*. Vol. 55, no. 6, p. 1467

Linder, S. & Alaiya, A. (2009) Serum efficacy biomarkers for oncology. *Biomark Med*. Vol. 3, no. 1, pp. 47-54

Lowery, A. & Han, Z. (2011) Assessment of tumor response to tyrosine kinase inhibitors. *Front Biosci*. Vol. 17, pp. 1996-2007

Ludwig, JA. & Weinstein, JN. (2005) Biomarkers in cancer staging, prognosis and treatment selection. *Nat Rev Cancer*, Vol. 5, no. 11, 845-856

Mahadevan, D., Plummer, R., Squires, MS., Rensvold, D., Kurtin, S., Pretzinger, C., Dragovich, T., Adams, J., Lock, V., Smith, DM., Von Hoff, D. & Calvert, H (2011) A phase I pharmacokinetic and pharmacodynamic study of AT7519, a cyclin-dependent kinase inhibitor in patients with refractory solid tumors. *Ann Oncol*. Vol. 22, no. 9, pp. 2137-2143

Mandrekar, SJ. & Sargent, DJ. (2010) Predictive biomarker validation in practice: lessons from real trials. *Clin Trials*, Vol. 7, no. 5, pp. 567-573

Mavroudis, D. (2010) Circulating cancer cells. *Ann Oncol*. Vol. 21, no. S7, pp. 95-100

Mehrara, E., Forssell-Aronsson, E. & Bernhardt, P. (2011) Objective assessment of tumor response to therapy based on tumor growth kinetics. *Br J Cancer*, Vol. 105, no. 5, pp. 682-686

Melichar, B. & Zezulova, M. (2011) The significance of altered gastrointestinal permeability in cancer patients. *Curr Opin Support Palliat Care*, Vol. 5, no. 1, pp. 47-54

Micha, D., Cummings, J., Shoemaker, A., Elmore, S., Foster, K., Greaves, M., Ward, T., Rosenberg, S., Dive, C. & Simpson, K. (2008) Circulating biomarkers of cell death after treatment with the BH-3 mimetic ABT-737 in a preclinical model of small-cell lung cancer. *Clin Cancer Res*. Vol. 14, no. 22, pp. 7304-7310

Mishra, A. & Verma, M. (2010) Cancer Biomarkers: Are We Ready for the Prime Time? *Cancers*, Vol. 2010, no. 2, pp. 190-208

Natori, S., Rust, C., Stadheim, LM., Srinivasan, A., Burgart, LJ. & Gores GJ. (2001) Hepatocyte apoptosis is a pathologic feature of human alcoholic hepatitis. *J Hepatol.* Vol. 34, no. 2, pp. 248-253

Olofsson, MH., Ueno, T., Pan, Y., Xu, R., Cai, F., van der Kuip, H., Muerdter, TE., Sonnenberg, M., Aulitzky, WE., Schwarz, S., Andersson, E., Shoshan, MC., Havelka, AM., Toi M. & Linder, S. (2007) Cytokeratin-18 is a useful serum biomarker for early determination of response of breast carcinomas to chemotherapy. *Clin Cancer Res.* Vol. 13, no. 11, pp. 3198-3206

Olofsson, MH., Cummings, J., Fayad, W., Brnjic, S., Herrmann, R., Berndtsson, M., Hodgkinson, C., Dean, E., Odedra, R., Wilkinson, RW., Mundt, KE., Busk, M., Dive, C. & Linder, S. (2009) Specific demonstration of drug-induced tumor cell apoptosis in human xenografts models using a plasma biomarker. *Cancer Biomark.* Vol. 5, no. 3, pp. 117-125

Ozturk, B., Coskun, U., Sancak, B., Yaman, E., Buyukberber, S. & Benekli, M. (2009) Elevated serum levels of M30 and M65 in patients with locally advanced head and neck tumors. *Int Immunopharmacol.* Vol. 9, no. 5, pp. 645–648

Padhani, AR. & Miles, KA. (2010) Multiparametric imaging of tumor response to therapy. *Radiology,* Vol. 256, no. 2, pp. 348-364

Pan, Y., Xu, R., Peach, M., Huang, CP., Branstetter, D., Novotny, W., Herbst, RS., Eckhardt, SG. & Holland, PM. (2011) Evaluation of pharmacodynamic biomarkers in a Phase 1a trial of dulanermin (rhApo2L/TRAIL) in patients with advanced tumors. *Br J Cancer,* Vol. 105, no. 12, pp. 1830-1838

Pantel, K. & Alix-Panabières, C. (2010) Circulating tumour cells in cancer patients: challenges and perspectives. *Trends Mol Med.* Vol. 16, no. 9, pp. 398-406

Paules, M., Casey, M., Williams, G., Swann, RS., Murphy, PS., Salazar, VM., Foose, D., Bailey, B. & Therasse, P. (2011) Recommendations for capture, validation and summarisation of data from studies using RECIST. *Eur J Cancer,* Vol. 47, no. 5, pp. 697-701

Perez-Soler, R. (2006) Rash as a surrogate marker for efficacy of epidermal growth factor receptor inhibitors in lung cancer. *Clin Lung Cancer,* Vol. 8, no. S1, pp. S7-14

De Petris, L., Brandén, E., Herrmann, R., Sanchez, BC., Koyi, H., Linderholm, B., Lewensohn, R., Linder, S. & Lehtiö, J. (2011) Diagnostic and prognostic role of plasma levels of two forms of cytokeratin 18 in patients with non-small-cell lung cancer. *Eur J Cancer,* Vol. 47, no. 1, pp. 131-137

Pichon, MF., Labroquère, M., Rezaï, K. & Lokiec, F. (2006) Variations of soluble fas and cytokeratin 18-Asp 396 neo-epitope in different cancers during chemotherapy. *Anticancer Res,* Vol. 26, no. 3B, pp. 2387-2392

Ross, JS., Torres-Mora, J., Wagle, N., Jennings, TA. & Jones, DM. (2010) Biomarker-based prediction of response to therapy for colorectal cancer: current perspective. *Am J Clin Pathol.* Vol. 134, no. 3, pp. 478-490

Roth, GA., Krenn, C., Brunner, M., Moser, B., Ploder, M., Spittler, A., Pelinka, L., Sautner, T., Wolner, E., Boltz-Nitulescu, G. & Ankersmit, HJ. (2004) Elevated serum levels of epithelial cell apoptosis-specific cytokeratin 18 neoepitope m30 in critically ill patients. *Shock,* Vol. 22, no. 3, pp. 218-220

Schellenberger, EA., Bogdanov, A Jr., Petrovsky, A., Ntziachristos, V., Weissleder, R. & Josephson, L. (2003) Optical imaging of apoptosis as a biomarker of tumor response to chemotherapy. *Neoplasia*, Vol. 5, no. 3, pp. 187-192

Schuell, B., Gruenberger, T., Kornek, GV., Dworan, N., Depisch, D., Lang, F., Schneeweiss, B. & Scheithauer, W. (2005) Side effects during chemotherapy predict tumor response in advanced colorectal cancer. *Br J Cancer*, Vol. 93, no. 7, pp. 744-748

Saad, ED., Katz, A., Hoff, PM. & Buyse, M. (2010) Progression-free survival as surrogate and as true end point: insights from the breast and colorectal cancer literature. *Ann Oncol*. Vol. 21, no. 1, pp. 7-12

Schutte, B., Henfling, M., Kölgen, W., Bouman, M., Meex, S., Leers, MP., Nap, M., Björklund, V., Björklund, P., Björklund, B., Lane, EB., Omary, MB., Jörnvall, H. & Ramaekers, FC. (2004) Keratin 8/18 breakdown and reorganization during apoptosis. *Exp Cell Res*. Vol. 297, no. 1, pp. 11-26

Schwarzenbach, H., Hoon, DS. & Pantel K. (2011) Cell-free nucleic acids as biomarkers in cancer patients. *Nat Rev Cancer*, Vol. 11, no. 6, pp. 426-437

Scott, LC., Evans, TR., Cassidy, J., Harden, S., Paul, J., Ullah, R., O'Brien, V. & Brown, R. (2009) Cytokeratin 18 in plasma of patients with gastrointestinal adenocarcinoma as a biomarker of tumor response. *Br J Cancer*, Vol. 101, no. 3, pp. 410-417

Shin, SJ., Jung, M., Jeung, HC., Kim, HR., Rha, SY., Roh, JK., Chung, HC. & Ahn, JB (2011) A phase I pharmacokinetic study of TSU-68 (a multiple tyrosine kinase inhibitor of VEGFR-2., FGF and PDFG) in combination with S-1 and oxaliplatin in metastatic colorectal cancer patients previously treated with chemotherapy. *Invest New Drugs*, 2011, in press.

Shtilbans, V., Wu, M. & Burstein, DE. (2010) Evaluation of apoptosis in cytologic specimens. *Diagn Cytopathol*. Vol. 38, no. 9, pp. 685-697

Steele, NL., Plumb, JA., Vidal, L., Tjørnelund, J., Knoblauch, P., Rasmussen, A., Ooi, CE., Buhl-Jensen, P., Brown, R., Evans, TR. & DeBono, JS. (2008) A phase 1 pharmacokinetic and pharmacodynamic study of the histone deacetylase inhibitor belinostat in patients with advanced solid tumors. *Clin Cancer Res*. Vol. 14, no. 3, pp. 804-810

Stieber, P., Dienemann, H., Hasholzner, U, Müller, C., Poley, S., Hofmann, K. & Fateh-Moghadam A. (1993) Comparison of cytokeratin fragment 19 (CYFRA 21-1), tissue polypeptide antigen (TPA) and tissue polypeptide specific antigen (TPS) as tumor markers in lung cancer. *Eur J Clin Chem Clin Biochem*. Vol. 31, no. 10, pp. 689–694

Stigbrand, T., Andres, C., Bellanger, L., Bishr Omary, M., et al. (1998). Epitope specificity of 30 monoclonal antibodies against cytokeratin antigens: the ISOBM TD5-1 Workshop. *Tumor Biol*. Vol. 19, no. 2, pp. 132-152

Stigbrand, T. (2001) The versatility of cytokeratins as tumor markers. *Tumor Biol*. Vol. 22, no. 1, pp. 1–3

Strnad, P., Windoffer, R. & Leube, RE. (2002) Induction of rapid and reversible cytokeratin filament network remodeling by inhibition of tyrosine phosphatases. *J Cell Sci*. Vol. 115, no. 21, pp. 4133-4148

Sundström, BE. & Stigbrand, TI. Cytokeratins and tissue polypeptide antigen. *Int J Biol Markers*, Vol. 9, no. 2, pp. 102–108

Therasse, P., Arbuck, SG., Eisenhauer, EA., Wanders, J., Kaplan, RS., Rubinstein, L., et al. (2009) New guidelines to evaluate the response to treatment in solid tumors.

European Organization for Research and Treatment of Cancer. *J Natl Cancer Inst.* Vol. 92, pp. 205–216

Le Tourneau, C., Faivre, S., Laurence, V., Delbaldo, C., Vera, K., Girre, V., Chiao, J., Armour, S., Frame, S., Green, SR., Gianella-Borradori, A., Diéras, V. & Raymond, E. (2010) Phase I evaluation of seliciclib (R-roscovitine)., a novel oral cyclin-dependent kinase inhibitor., in patients with advanced malignancies. *Eur J Cancer*, Vol. 46, no. 18, pp. 3243-3250

Ueno, T., Toi, M., Bivén, K., Bando, H., Ogawa, T. & Linder, S. (2003) Measurement of an apoptosis product in the sera of breast cancer patients. *Eur J Cancer*, Vol. 39, no. 6, pp. 769–774

Ulukaya, E., Yilmaztepe, A., Akgoz, S., Akgoz, S., Linder, S. & Karadag, M. (2007) The levels of caspase-cleaved cytokeratin 18 are elevated in serum from patients with lung cancer and helpful to predict the survival. *Lung Cancer*, Vol. 56, no. 3, pp. 399–404

Ulukaya, E., Karaagac, E., Ari, F., Arzu, Y., Oral, AY., Adim, SB., Tokullugil, AH. & Evrensell, T. (2011) Chemotherapy increases caspase-cleaved cytokeratin 18 in the serum of breast cancer patients. *Radiol Oncol.* Vol. 45, no. 2, pp. 116-122

Ward, TH., Cummings, J., Dean, E., Greystoke, A., Hou, JM., Backen, A., Ranson, M. & Dive C. (2008) Biomarkers of apoptosis. *Br J Cancer*, Vol. 99, no. 6, pp. 841-846

Weber, K., Osborn, M., Moll, R.., Wiklund, B. & Lüning, B. (1984). Tissue polypeptide antigen (TPA) is related to the non-epidermal keratins 8, 18 and 19 typical of simple and non-squamous epithelia: re-evaluation of a human tumor marker. *EMBO J.* Vol. 3, no. 11, pp. 2707-2714

Weber, WA. (2009) Assessing tumor response to therapy. J Nucl Med. Vol. 50, no. S1, pp. 1S-10S

Wittenburg, LA. & Gustafson, DL. (2011) Optimizing preclinical study design in oncology research. *Chem Biol Interact.* Vol. 190, no. 2-3, pp. 73-78

Wolff, HA., Daldrup, B., Jung, K., Overbeck, T., Hennies, S., Matthias, C., Hess, CF., Roedel, RM. & Christiansen, H. (2011) High-grade acute organ toxicity as positive prognostic factor in adjuvant radiation and chemotherapy for locally advanced head and neck cancer. *Radiology*, Vol. 258, no. 3, pp. 864-871

Yagmur, E., Trautwein, C., Leers, MP., Gressner, AM. & Tacke, F. (2007) Elevated apoptosis-associated cytokeratin 18 fragments (CK18Asp386) in serum of patients with chronic liver diseases indicate hepatic and biliary inflammation. *Clin Biochem.* Vol. 40, no. 9-10, pp. 651-655

Yaman, E., Coskun, U., Sancak, B., Buyukberber, S., Ozturk, B. & Benekli, M. (2010) Serum M30 levels are associated with survival in advanced gastric carcinoma patients. *Int Immunopharmacol.* Vol. 10, no. 7, pp. 719-722

Zhao, B., Schwartz, LH. & Larson, SM. (2009) Imaging surrogates of tumor response to therapy: anatomic and functional biomarkers. *J Nucl Med.* Vol. 50, no. 2, pp. 239-249

Zong, WX. & Thompson, CB. (2006) Necrotic death as a cell fate. *Genes Dev.* Vol. 20, no. 1, pp. 1-15